Physician Communication

Physician Communication

Connecting with Patients, Peers, and the Public

TERRY L. SCHRAEDER, MD

Clinical Associate Professor
Warren Alpert Medical School of Brown University
Providence, Rhode Island, USA

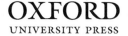

OXFORD
UNIVERSITY PRESS

OXFORD
UNIVERSITY PRESS

Oxford University Press is a department of the University of Oxford. It furthers
the University's objective of excellence in research, scholarship, and education
by publishing worldwide. Oxford is a registered trade mark of Oxford University
Press in the UK and certain other countries.

Published in the United States of America by Oxford University Press
198 Madison Avenue, New York, NY 10016, United States of America.

Library of Congress Cataloging-in-Publication Data
Names: Schraeder, Terry L., author.
Title: Physician communication : connecting with patients, peers, and the public /
Terry L. Schraeder.
Description: New York : Oxford University Press, 2019. |
Includes bibliographical references and index.
Identifiers: LCCN 2019006313 | ISBN 9780190882440
Subjects: | MESH: Physician-Patient Relations | Communication
Classification: LCC R690 | NLM W 62 | DDC 610.73/72069—dc23
LC record available at https://lccn.loc.gov/2019006313

1 3 5 7 9 8 6 4 2

Printed by Integrated Books International, United States of America

Contents

Foreword

Like the rest of us, physicians as communicators fall along a wide spectrum of capability, sensitivity, and technical savvy. A few are compellingly effective in reaching their audience, and some are ineffective in or even oblivious to registering the impact of their words and accompanying actions. Enjoying the rare advantage of a successful career as a medical journalist, leading a decade later to earning a degree in medicine that combines clinical practice with academic responsibilities, Dr. Terry L. Schraeder has written an engaging, informed, and instructive volume on communication. Primarily directed to helping physicians in their contacts with patients, families, colleagues, the public, and the media, her eminently readable and well-researched volume is also of practical use to nurses, executives, and public affairs and development staff in medical environments and well beyond. Most of the insights and recommendations offered can benefit virtually anyone who wants to be more effective in getting important information across to another individual or group.

Focusing on face-to-face communication, Chapter 1 discusses patients' needs for clarity, some of the barriers that muddle it, and ways to overcome those barriers not only verbally but also through awareness of the "body English" of participants in the dialogue. The importance of the physician as a role model is underscored, particularly in helping shape attitudes and resulting communications of younger colleagues as well as in influencing the sensitivity and responsiveness of others in the hospital and office.

Chapter 2 reflects extensive research on available digital communication resources and their utility, advantages, and potential disadvantages. Offering sensible advice on how to avoid becoming overwhelmed by the plethora of programs offered and the massive input received from even sparse use of that cornucopia, Dr. Schraeder makes enough sense of this rapidly growing and diverse digital world not only to calm anxieties of older physicians but also to encourage its more efficient use by the profession's younger and more digitally facile cohort. Sound advice is offered on using digital media effectively in doctor–patient dialogue and in avoiding drowning in the torrent of useless input.

Public speaking and presentation are approached in Chapter 3. These may be the touchiest subjects of this book because one's experience as a listener commonly suggests that a multitude of speakers seem to feel they do rather well as is, or don't care to know how to become more effective. Many helpful details will benefit delivery for the physician. Beyond content, practical advice (in the realm of common sense that needs articulation but is often ignored) is laid out with respect to dress, posture, eye contact, effective visuals, and other details that encourage speakers to contemplate needs and perceptions of their audiences. That awareness is not easy to achieve, but it might be encouraged by reviewing one's delivery, not in a mirror at home, but rather by scrutinizing one's recent performance on a TV news or discussion program. Advice for the novice: don't be surprised—"Good heavens! Is that me?"

Chapter 4 delves into the traditional media arena, where many physicians seem to feel mistakenly that their professional expertise is sufficient to satisfy contact with the media and the public beyond, just as it generally may be sufficient in their contact with medical peers. The expertise of sound public relations and communications experts is neither to be distained nor avoided. They know better what influences the lay public as well as the challenges of getting meaningful information to the public despite the barrage of information and countervailing half-truths that bathe them through

TV. Physicians may fail to realize that the legitimate needs of media differ from those of interprofessional communications and that can lead to problems including an important message being sullied or ending up "lost on the cutting room floor." Whether through an op-ed for the local newspaper, a professional comment on radio or TV, or a description of an event at the hospital, happy or not, getting across important points calls for thoughtful advance preparation, often practice in delivery, and careful control of both delivery and content.

To sum it up, Dr. Schraeder has used her rich experience of several decades as an active medical journalist, practicing clinician, and teacher to create a detailed and thoughtful compendium characterizing the challenges of communication by physicians with patients, colleagues, the public, and the media. She offers workable opportunities to increase effectiveness in conveying what physicians feel is important and in gaining sensitivity and responsiveness to the needs of their diverse and sometimes vulnerable audiences.

Mitchell T. Rabkin, MD

Professor of Medicine, Harvard Medical School

CEO Emeritus, Boston's Beth Israel Hospital (1966–1996)

Preface

Communicare: To Communicate

On March 9, 1929, the *Saturday Evening Post* published an iconic cover illustration of an elderly doctor placing his stethoscope on the chest of a doll held by a little girl. The famous painting, "Doctor and Doll" by Norman Rockwell, depicted a much simpler and innocent time, but it may also serve as an allegory to the world of physician communication. In looking at the early-twentieth-century scene, one sees the grandfatherly figure taking the time to recognize what is important to the patient—her doll—and using it to establish an emotional bridge.

In 1989, I met Dr. Donald Campbell, a physician who served as a model for Norman Rockwell. The family doctor was depicted with a child in another famous Rockwell painting, "Before the Shot." Dr. Campbell was retiring from his solo practice in Lenox, Massachusetts, and I was working as a medical journalist. In writing a story about his life, I followed the 83-year-old practitioner as he made his last house calls. It was clear that patients respected and appreciated him. I asked him what the most important aspect of taking care of patients was, and I will never forget his response: "Patients need us to listen to them."

Physician–patient communication is, after all, human-to-human communication; establishing a bond and listening are just two of the essential elements in building trust and understanding—the foundations of communication. But today there is much we need to learn when it comes to facilitating the exchange of information, providing psychosocial support, ensuring shared decision-making, translating complex information, resolving controversies with sound science, and the myriad of goals we have as physician communicators with patients, peers, and the public.

While most of our communication is with patients, we increasingly find ourselves communicating with family members, caregivers, students, residents, colleagues, patient advocates, researchers, insurance agencies, bosses, board members, the public, and even at times journalists. What we are communicating, where we are communicating, and with whom we are communicating are continually changing and expanding—and with ever more electronic technologies, from electronic medical records and emails to online forums, video conferencing, and other high-tech systems available to us. All of this makes how we communicate even more important to our success.

Although we may not possess the journalistic and writing skills of Atul Gawande, the policy platform of the former US Surgeon General Vivek Murthy, or the articulate discourse of Anthony Fauci, the director of the National Institute of Allergy and Infectious Diseases (NIAID), much less the leisurely patient visits of the Norman Rockwell era, we can no doubt learn and benefit from improved communication skills. Today, we may watch pediatric neurosurgeon Tony Adkins dancing with his patients on YouTube (making a more animated and modern emotional connection than Norman Rockwell), or we may find ourselves emailing with patients or Skyping with peers; it is clear that the world of communication for physicians has changed in many ways since the creation of the "Doctor and Doll" painting.

What does it mean to be a physician communicator?

The word "communicate" is defined by the *Merriam-Webster Dictionary* as, "to convey knowledge or information" and "to transmit information, thought, or feeling so that it is satisfactorily received or understood." The *Oxford English Dictionary* describes communication as the ability to "succeed in conveying one's ideas or in evoking understanding in others." The origin of the word communicate comes from the Latin word *communicare* meaning "to make common" and "share, impart or inform." Now, maybe more than ever, it is both relevant and important for physicians to think about how they communicate with their patients and in public so they can develop a bond and inform their audience. After all, with each sentence we speak, we are conveying a message and continually negotiating our relationship with our audience, according to Steven Pinker, author of *The Language Instinct*.

The origin of the word communicate also comes from Latin *communicatus* meaning "to impart information" and "to transmit a feeling" and *communis* meaning "common, public, and general." The premise of communication rests on finding and sharing something in common between two parties, another critical element in the translation of clinical information. Dr. Tim Johnson, the former ABC News television medical editor, was an excellent physician communicator for the public because he translated information into language, images, and stories that the audience could understand and relate to. For decades, he informed, educated, and calmed the public with explanations of complex and breaking medical stories on television. He, like other physician communicators such as Jerome Groopman (author of *How Doctors Think* and other books), Siddhartha Mukherjee (*The Emperor of All Maladies* and *The Gene*) and the late Richard Selzer (*The Doctor Stories* and other books), was a master storyteller—using common language to describe observations and insights into the human condition.

As physicians, the way we listen, observe, reflect, intuit, and ask questions, as well as the words we use to describe, translate or explain, are all relevant and essential; our specific tone, volume, articulation, and emphasis contribute to how we communicate. Of course, nonverbal communication underscores a significant part of all communication; the body language cues we transmit and observe are essential. Our intention underscores our communication; but miscommunication, whether it is verbal or nonverbal, can obstruct our objectives. Whether we are speaking face to face or using electronic technology, the human qualities of our communication skills can and should be identified, evaluated, and amended as necessary. Whether it is finding an emotional connection or a common language, deciphering our audience's needs, or just honing compassionate awareness and our language skills, it is part of our job as physicians to make sure we know how to listen and how to be heard.

Perhaps we need to go back as far as Aristotle, who believed that the development of rhetoric was an art worthy of systematic and scientific study. The ancient Greek philosopher and scientist identified the critical elements of a good communicator: ethos (character), pathos (personal connection), and logos (words). We might also benefit from remembering the basic tenets of journalists who share so many of the same skills as physicians, such as listening, observation, recording, and translation; we need to remember the "who, what, when, where, why, and how" of modern-day physician communications in the twenty-first century.

We could certainly learn from behavioral science and other disciplines about the knowledge and understanding of human interactions as well as how to decipher, transmit, and adapt effective techniques of human contact, relationships, and interdependence. Being aware of ourselves, our physical settings, and any communication barriers, as well as our eye contact, language, mannerisms, voice, appearance, and posture—and how they all affect the patient's perception of our communication, competency, and care—is pertinent to our success as clinicians.

The Patient Protection and Affordable Care Act's emphasis on improved primary care and the adoption of patient-centered medical homes has also intensified interest in patient-centered communication skills. Unfortunately, despite several decades of published research on the importance of physician communication skills, many physicians, once they are in practice, receive little if any specific training, including feedback and exercise of skills, in this area. We need help not only at the bedside with patients and at the lecture podium with distracted audiences but also with our keyboards, computer screens, and other electronic modes of communication. With the ever-changing demands of the healthcare field and its increased quantity and complexity of information and individual interactions, as well as the various new roles and responsibilities we are assuming in education, business, media, and government, we need more insight and guidance than ever.

Glaring omissions from the historical Rockwell paintings are computer screens, electronic medical records, time-limited office visits, insurance forms, malpractice suits, cultural and language differences, misaligned expectations, continuing medical education hours, distracted audiences of residents, board recertification tests, Skype video teleconferences, mountains of paperwork, miles of emails, uncoordinated specialists' consultations, and a waiting room full of anxious and sick patients requesting tests and treatments that may not be medically warranted. Missing from the Rockwell renditions are our Internet-informed patients with strong opinions about their diagnosis and treatment and angry patients complaining, often appropriately, that their wait times are too long and their visits are too short. Can we glean lessons from the slower paced personal physician of the past to help us navigate our modern moving landscape and become better physician communicators in a variety of different settings? Can we draw from other academic and professional disciplines, such as education, media, business, theology, theater, law, and education, for help? Can we look at the specific words and vocabulary we use and the biases and preconceived notions we bear to our interactions and how they are hindering us?

In my own work as a physician, medical educator, and journalist, I have observed many physicians struggling with their own communication skills. I have taught courses and given presentations on communication skills for physicians and scientists. I, along with my colleagues, have received wonderful as well as less than glowing online reviews from patients. During my seminars, I am asked the following questions by physicians: "Why don't my patients like me?"; "How can I make my research more understandable to lay audiences?"; "I know how to provide excellent care but how can I better connect with my patients?"; "Where should I look when I am interviewed on camera?"; "What mistakes do you see in my public speaking and presentations?"; and "Should I use social media as a doctor?"

I have conducted my professional life at the crossroads of clinical medicine, medical education, journalism, and mass communications. As a medical internist and a writer, I have worked as the Graduate Medical Education Editor at the *New England Journal of Medicine* and on television and in newspapers and magazines as a medical journalist. My work has appeared in the *New England Journal of Medicine*, the *Boston Globe*, ABC News, *60 Minutes*, *Good Morning America*, WBUR-NPR, the *Harvard Neiman Reports*, *Science Editor*, and other publications. I take care of patients at Mount Auburn Hospital in Cambridge, Massachusetts and am Clinical Associate Professor at the Warren Alpert Medical School at Brown University in Providence, Rhode Island, where I direct the scholarly concentration, Physician as Communicator, and a course on medical journalism.

In writing this book, I have witnessed my own evolution of knowledge and behavior in this area. I believe I have become more sensitive, informed, observant, and articulate; the result has been an improvement in my own awareness and performance in patient interactions and presentations. I hope that while reading this book, you will have your own transformation and improvement in many of the different areas of communication you encounter within the profession of medicine.

Over the course of my career, I have interviewed many physicians considered expert physician communicators, from historical figures such as cardiac surgeon Michael DeBakey and US Surgeon General C. Everett Koop to current leaders such as the director of the NIAID, Anthony Fauci and the director of the National

Institutes of Health, Francis Collins. Throughout the work on this book, I have gathered advice from expert communicators as well as data and lessons from the science of communications. As a working physician and journalist, I have spent many years navigating and discovering necessary communication and interpersonal skills in clinical settings, academic institutions, and the media.

Throughout this book, I aim to share what I know and to guide you to those who will teach us more about this important subject. I have developed a system I use to teach presentation and communication skills called "MACY." I will write more about various approaches and techniques throughout this book, but here is a brief introduction to MACY—and I will use it to tell you why I wrote this book. My MACY approach can be used before any presentation or communication interaction.

M is for mission. What is the mission or reason for this presentation or interaction? You need to know your goals and purpose before you start so that when it is over, you will know if you succeeded. You will want to articulate clearly to yourself why you are seeing this patient, speaking to a colleague, or presenting at a medical conference—or writing a book. What is your overall goal? Why is it important that your communication is the best that it can be and this interaction goes well? Will improved communication help you take better care of your patients, receive a promotion after your presentation, help to publish and acknowledge your research, evaluate an employee, educate the audience on an important matter, or inform the public by speaking to a journalist?

My mission in writing this book is to help the individuals working in a profession that I dearly love and deeply respect, who are in need of better communication skills. If I can help you communicate better, then I know that your important work as a clinician, researcher, public health expert, or scientist will be more accessible and more effective.

A is for audience. Who is your audience (or the patient in front of you) and what do they need from you? What do they already know and what don't they know? How can you listen, observe, inform, educate, enlighten, and help? What are the audiences' expectations, questions, thoughts, and desires? What is the patient's mood? What is the audience's understanding of your message and your work? How can you best connect and communicate with them?

My audience for this book is you—the health care practitioners who need help communicating with their patients one to one despite barriers of electronics, time limitations, and other problems; the medical educators who need help teaching distracted students or residents; and the scientists who need to improve their presentation skills or their connection to the media in order to translate and publicize their complex work to others.

C is for content. What is the actual content of your presentation or words of intercourse of communication? Are you knowledgeable and prepared? Is your presentation complete and organized? Is your research and writing educational and engaging? Have you reviewed the material as much as you can? Have you predicted and prepared for tough questions your audience may ask? Have you written brief statements of facts or bulleted important points you need to make?

My content for this book is based on important published research, articles, and interviews, as well as my own work, expertise, and observations as a physician communicator. I have compiled, edited, translated, and written this information for you in a clear, thoughtful, referenced, and relevant manner so that you can learn new skills and how to adapt them for your own professional and personal use.

Y is for you. You are the communicator preparing for the interaction. Why are you the best person for this interaction? Are you calm, prepared, well-rested, and confident? Are you ready to utilize all that you have at your disposal to make this moment of communication the best that it can be? Imagine that it is over before you begin—how did it go?

My "you" in this case is me (since I am writing the book). I will draw on resources and my own experience in communications to present knowledge on what makes for effective information exchange in the current healthcare environment. I hope to teach you how to be the best communicator you can be.

It is very possible that physicians in the past thought little about any of this before they interacted with others. But then again, they likely had their own strategies and practices, consciously and unconsciously, to connect to their patients and to larger groups—certainly the doctors depicted by Norman Rockwell did. After all, the theme of this book is defining and discovering how you, today's physician, can best connect to your patients, peers, the public, and the press so that you and your message are satisfactorily received and understood. Many of the different settings, types, and methods of communication I will present require different skill sets and different approaches and emphasis, but there will also be many common themes between the different modalities that underscore the intricacies, nuances, and basics of human-to-human interactions.

This book is divided into four chapters: Face-to-Face Communication, Digital Communication, Public Speaking and Presentations, and Traditional Media. Each of these may help you in situations you may find yourself in with patients, students and residents, family members, caregivers, peers, your community, the press, and the public. I hope that the information and advice will prompt you to examine, analyze, and improve your skills in the art and science of physician communications. Norman Rockwell may have painted endearing pictures of doctors in clinical settings, but if we are to look back and learn from the spirit of these nostalgic images, we have to start by evaluating ourselves and being honest about our own success and failure as well as our current constraints and responsibilities using all the modes of communication available today. We need specific skills to adapt as well as global and

institutional direction and support. I hope this book will provide
the information and help you need.

Think like a wise man but communicate in the language of the
people.

—W. B. Yeats

The biggest communication problem is that we do not listen to
understand. We listen to reply.

—Gabriel Garcia Marquez

The patient will never care how much you know, until they
know how much you care.

—Terry Canale, American Academy of Orthopaedic Surgeons

Acknowledgments

No author can write a book without all of the important people, experiences, and resources available along the way. I thank everyone who offered their support. Your encouragement, guidance, and friendship kept me working and bringing this idea to fruition.

Thank you to the individuals in medicine, journalism, and my personal life who have mentored, taught, and inspired me in big and small ways, including Charlie Hatem, Tim Johnson, the late John Harrington, Jeffrey M. Drazen, Julie Ingelfinger, Tad Campion, Roger Sergel, Roman DeSanctis, Mitch Rabkin, Jerry Kassirer, Marcia Angell, the late Arnold S. Rehlman, Jerry Groopman, Allan Tunkel, Thais Mather, Brian Clyne, Len Mermel, Jeffrey Borkan, Reverend Rebecca Spencer, Rabbi Leslie Y. Gutterman, Robert Naparstek, Fred Sullivan Jr., Wonbo Woo, Anna Delamerced, Nils Bruzelius, Emily Green, Sarah Freeman, Judith Bentkover, Jim Baird, Jen Mellen, Miho Cha, Mary Cappello, Shelly Roth, Carl Freedman, Stephen Kurkjian, Christine Montross, LuAnn Cserr, Karen Schiffman, Malaga Baldi, Jill Friedlander, Charlotte Raymond, Michael Gross at The Authors Guild, and so many others.

Much of this book is a product of the lectures and workshops I continue to present at the Warren Alpert Medical School of Brown University and other institutions. Thank you to all the students and faculty affiliated with the Executive Masters in Healthcare Leadership Program, the Primary Care-Population Medicine Program, and the Program in Educational and Faculty Development at Brown University. Thank you to the *NEJM* editor-in-chief Jeffrey M. Drazen and his assistant Pam Miller for inviting me to speak every year to the medical students at the *New England Journal of Medicine*. Thank you to Drs. James May and Paul Duncan for honoring me with the Dr. Ed Bierman Lectureship for my talk,

"Physician Communications in the 21st Century." I thank all of the individuals and audiences I have had the great opportunity to meet, teach, and, most important, learn from.

At Oxford University Press, I am so appreciative of Andrea Knobloch at Oxford University Press who was helpful and encouraging from day one; and wonderful Annie Sanchez who shined as a new editor at OUP with her superb edits and ideas.

Thank you to the John D. Rockefeller, Jr. Library at Brown University ("the Rock") and to our public libraries, particularly the Peace Dale, Cranston Central, and East Providence Public Libraries in Rhode Island and the Weston Library in Massachusetts. Our public libraries are jewels of refuge and knowledge. May they continue to be enriching, warm, welcoming, and quiet.

To my dear friends, Deb Kroll, Merle Goldstein, Mary Hedahl, Amy Saltonstall, Vicki Saltonstall, Vicky Davison, Jen Mellen, Doug Laird, Christine Nassikas, and Meg Magee: thank you for always being there for me. To Ann Williams, an incredible second mother, mentor, and friend. To my brother and true friend, Scott. To my husband and life partner, Rick Terek, thank you. For my mom and dad, now both gone—their love and lessons live on in me and in this book.

I wrote this book to help those working in the profession of medicine—a profession I deeply admire and believe in. My hope is that this book furthers the discussion about the importance of communication for all of us.

The three most important lessons I learned while writing this book are:

1. Listening is a physical exam skill.
2. We can only truly communicate when we are fully present.
3. Our care improves as our communication improves.

Terry L. Schraeder, MD
2019

Physician Communication

1

Face-to-Face Communication

The biggest problem in communication is the illusion that it has taken place.

—George Bernard Shaw

I've learned that people will forget what you said, people will forget what you did, but they will never forget how you made them feel.

—Maya Angelou

Introduction

There I was in the clinic, toe-to-toe with a 75-year-old woman yelling at me, "I need steroid pills!" She had a patch of four small hives on her right arm. She also had diabetes and osteoporosis. I sat down and asked her if she would like to sit down, too. I listened, asked questions, and tried to be empathic and explain in reasonable and clear language why oral steroids were not medically indicated and, furthermore, carried risks for her. Her voice escalated, "I don't have a car. They told me I would get steroids. I live on the third floor with no air conditioning. This rash is going to erupt and get in my system if you don't give me steroids." I kept thinking to myself, "I am a doctor and am currently writing a book about physician communications, and this interaction is not going so well."

During the course of writing this book, I would like to say that all of my face-to-face communications, especially with patients, have been perfect. Unfortunately, they have not. Before starting this project, I thought I had little room for improvement in this area. I was wrong. Through my research, study, and interviewing of experts for this book, I have learned much, and thankfully watched my own interactions and communication skills improve.

Are people born natural communicators? While some individuals are particularly gifted at these skills, for the most part people learn their communication skills, and how to improve them, through observation, training, courses, books, practice, and feedback. The good news is that it is possible to learn new techniques and methods to help you improve in order to have more positive therapeutic interactions with your patients. Just by becoming aware of the many issues of communication and acknowledging your own style and skills, you may augment all of your interactions. Also, it is possible not only to learn and adapt new skills but also to teach trainees how to do this. If we can enhance and deepen discussions with our patients and make them authentic and spontaneous—not forced, artificial, or formulaic—and remember the reasons we became doctors in the first place, we can ensure better relationships with our patients and hope for the future of our profession.

The eminent physician Roman W. DeSanctis taught at Harvard Medical School and practiced cardiology for 60 years. We can learn much from this brilliant caring clinician and authentic communicator. For years, he has spoken and written about the importance of deepening our connection to patients and always treating them with respect, dignity, and patience. Any discussion of patient communications should start with Dr. DeSanctis's five pillars of medicine, which he calls the basis of his decades-long professional and moral practice.[1]

FACE-TO-FACE COMMUNICATION 3

Five Pillars for the Practice of Medicine

1. The patient should always come first in the life of a doctor.
2. In any situation, and at any time, weigh all of the information in hand and always try to do that which is best for the patient.
3. As the Golden Rule applies to life, so it applies in the practice of medicine.
4. Be a friend to your patients, as well as a caregiver.
5. Always demonstrate your humanity with honesty, sincerity, and empathy.

Source: Dr. Roman DeSanctis, Harvard Medical School.

Remembering why we wanted to become doctors in the first place may be the most important step in improving our communication with patients. We know that our inherent values and ultimate life motives are the foundation of our missions as doctors. Unfortunately, in our current medical climate of extremely high-speed, computer-dependent, robotic, and seemingly drive-through doctor visits, the intimacy and satisfaction of caring for our patients is often diminished. We may not even be asking how we can best communicate and connect with our patients or even why we should.

On another day while writing this book, a 90-year-old man with a draining and purulent wound on his leg is shouting at me, "Why do I need IV antibiotics?" I calmly respond, "Because we don't want the infection in your leg to spread to your bloodstream." "Oh, you mean sepsis?" he snarls and then snaps at the nurses that he needs to go to the bathroom. A nurse cheerfully helps him down the hall to the bathroom in his wheelchair. A few minutes later, he is smiling and says, "This place is just terrific." Thank God for the nurses and of course for bathroom breaks. We start his intravenous antibiotic medication, and thankfully, he clinically improves.

Patients can be happy with you one minute and unhappy the next—and sometimes it depends on something as simple as a bathroom break (for you or for the patient) or plumping the patient's pillow. But sometimes it is much more complicated. As physicians we have to step back, be patient, assess what is going on with each particular situation, and continue to treat each patient thoughtfully and respectfully. At times working with patients is an emotional volatile rollercoaster. We as physicians have to ride it out. Whether we are working in the intensive care unit (ICU) or the emergency department (ED) or in an outpatient or urgent care setting, the need for optimal communication is paramount. After all, we are here to help make the patients as comfortable, informed, and cared for as possible.

An hour later, a 30-year-old patient with miliaria (heat rash) on his inner thighs loudly complains to me that our 30 minutes together (when I listened to his history, examined him, answered his questions, and explained my diagnosis and proposed treatment) was a waste of his time. I thought it had all gone so well. I was left to wonder what I could have done differently. Later I learned the patient had waited for more than two hours to see me. He was mad long before I saw him. If I had noticed his mood from his body language and activity (pacing the room, using his cell phone, and not wanting to sit down or be examined on the exam table), I could have softened my own approach, apologized for the wait, and listened to and acknowledged his anger long before he stormed out.

As a physician, you no doubt have your own stories of unhappy, frustrated, or angry patients, including the patients who disagree with you about not prescribing antibiotics or narcotics or the ones who want a magnetic resonance imaging (MRI) study after two days of knee pain. Most patients just need to hear a thoughtful explanation of their diagnosis, thorough answers to their questions, and your medical reasoning and therapeutic recommendations. But it is true that on any given day, seeing many different patients with a myriad of different problems can bring up various challenging discussions and situations. Your ability to make a human connection to each patient will always improve your communication and ultimately your care—knowing that each conversation may be as diverse and varied as the patients themselves.

Can we learn how to take care of patients and at the same time always have a respectful, positive, and therapeutic interaction together? Can we provide excellent care despite the time limitations we are under and the computer screen between us, and make sure the patients are happy with their care and their doctors? Are there natural physician communicators among us? Why are some excellent clinicians so good at this and others so inept when it comes to interacting with patients? How can we deepen our connection to patients and enhance their experience and ours by improving our skills?

First, our success at face-to-face communications with patients is highly dependent on understanding our patients, ourselves, and the intricacies and nuances of clinical communication. We no doubt must acknowledge, establish, and strengthen our human interconnection to each individual patient. Despite the ever-increased mechanization and computer-driven clinical sphere, we still work in a very personal intimate setting with humans often going through life-changing moments. Ultimately, we need to have humility, patience, and compassion both with our patients and with ourselves. After all, we practice our profession in an environment where pain, stress, and suffering are common and where so many factors are beyond our control. These factors range from the patients' experience before they see us to their expectations for the visit; from their health literacy to their individual social and cultural contexts; from the physical space we see them in to the physical spaces they live in; and from their opinions and past interactions with our profession to our own understanding and ability to connect emotionally. Underlying any attempt at improving our connection to our patients is the mission inside the exam room to make sure our profession remains a public service helping patients and not a business with a bottom line. Unfortunately, we as physicians come together daily with our patients in a virtual landmine of strained and tense interactions, in a profession in turmoil, and with changing patient expectations along with our own high levels of frustration and emotional burnout.

Think about your own interactions with patients at the most basic level. Have you knocked on a patient's door expecting to have a wonderfully therapeutic session and offer your services, only to be shut down with a negative reception? Or have you asked a patient what you thought was a clinically important and straightforward question and received an uninformative response or, worse, one filled with a few disrespectful comments? Have you thought you were giving a full explanation of a diagnosis only to be derailed by the patient's disagreement and oral history of their distrust of physicians? On the other hand, how often have you listened to friends complain about rude and dismissive physicians? Or have you heard a relative or an acquaintance tell a story about receiving bad news from an abrasive and condescending doctor? The litany of complaints about physicians' communication skills, behavior, and professional etiquette is long and sometimes seems to be getting longer.

We may all have stories of clinical situations in which the emotional tenor of the room escalates as our communication plummets; when the supportive caring environment we hoped for crumbles before our eyes, our effectiveness is weakened, and hope for a therapeutic interaction is somewhat, if not completely, curtailed. The disconnection between physicians and patients is often more than evident; and while the patience and emotional stamina of all parties are tested, both soon realize the communication is not going well. We wish we could rewind the scenario and start again. Of course, as physicians and as patients, we want to avoid these miscommunications and be able to relate, listen, and connect so that we can successfully demonstrate and achieve what we went into medicine to do in the first place—care for the patient. But how do we do this?

We know that learning and improving our face-to-face communication skills should help us support our patients and ourselves and diminish uncomfortable, unproductive, or, at worst, adversarial interactions. Inherently we know that if we hone our skills of listening, respect, expressing concern, sharing, and collaborating, then our care of our patients and their clinical outcomes will be optimized. Our backgrounds, personal experiences, societal stereotypes, and cultural contexts all have an impact on our decisions and actions. We also need to know that our implicit or unconscious biases affect our judgments and assessments of patients and situations. We need to learn how to limit the negative influences that limit our abilities to connect and care for patients.

Underlying all of it is the patients' need to retain their agency. In social science, agency is the capacity of individuals to be respected and to make their own decisions. Patients need information, support, and guidance and as long as they are competent and not in an emergency situation, they need to make (or help make) their own decisions. Patients are ultimately in charge of their bodies and their lives. They should always be treated with dignity, reverence, humanity, humility, and sincerity. We who work in healthcare organizations must ensure that our patients' agency is protected, encouraged, and assured no matter who they are or the structure or circumstances of the environment.

Why We Should Care

Once, while presenting a physician communications lecture at a medical conference, I was taken aback when a surgeon raised his hand and asked me, "My clinical outcomes are great, why should I care about my communication skills?" His question seemed to represent a past sentiment from a previously paternalistic time of medicine. But today, fortunately, we live and work in a patient-centered world of medicine, and the attitudes of many physicians and healthcare institutions have changed. Our interpersonal skills and relationships with patients are a priority, or at least they should be. My answer to the surgeon on that day was, "Along with our established clinical outcomes, which are still imperative, our communication is now an additional outcome to measure." I know this to be true because how we act, think, and talk as physicians are central to a patient's experience. After all, our communication affects not only the patient's clinical course, satisfaction, and behaviors but also our own rankings, ratings, reimbursement, burnout, liability, and healthcare costs according to several decades of research on physician–patient communications and institutions such as the Cleveland Clinic Center for Excellence in Healthcare Communications.[2]

Beginning more than a decade ago, The Joint Commission that accredits more than 21,000 healthcare organizations and programs in the United States, concluded that communication problems in medicine are one of the most common causes of sentinel events.[3] A "sentinel event" is defined as any unanticipated event resulting in death or serious physical or psychological injury to a patient, not related to the natural course of the patient's illness.[4] The Joint Commission now recommends an approach to communicating health information that "encompasses language needs, individual understanding, and cultural and other communication issues" and provides information and resources on The Joint Commission's Health Equity Portal.[5] For more than a decade, other academic institutions and accrediting boards of medicine have defined, endorsed, or required training and demonstrated competency in physician communication and interpersonal skills. Those organizations include the American Association of Medical Colleges, American Medical Association, American Board of Medical Specialties, Liaison Committee on Medical Education, and Institutes of Medicine.

Patient Satisfaction Surveys

For several years, the Centers for Medicare and Medicaid Services (CMS) have queried hospitalized adult patients about their care with Hospital Consumer Assessment of Healthcare Providers and Systems (HCAHPS) surveys.[6] The 32-item survey is conducted by mail or phone two to forty-two days after the patient is discharged. It captures the patients' unique perspectives on hospital care for the purpose of providing the public, and the government, with comparable information on hospital quality, including how well doctors and nurses communicate. Patients who have been recently hospitalized, with any type of payer plan, are randomly surveyed about the communication skills of their caregivers, along with questions about pain management, cleanliness, quietness, and overall ratings of the hospital. The HCAHPS survey includes questions such as, "Did your doctor explain things in a way you could understand?"; "Did your doctor listen to you?"; "Did your doctor treat you with courtesy and respect?" Hospitals who receive low scores on the HCAHPS survey can lose money through the Inpatient Prospective Payment System (IPPS) annual payment provisions. The incentive for IPPS hospitals to improve patient experience of care was further endorsed and strengthened by the Patient Protection and Affordable Care Act of 2010, which specifically included HCAHPS performance in the calculation of the value-based incentive payment in the Hospital Value-Based Purchasing program. About four thousand hospitals participate in HCAHPS, and more than three million patients complete the survey each year.[6] Since 2008, HCAHPS has allowed valid comparisons to be made across hospitals locally, regionally, and nationally.

The results from these surveys have prompted hospitals to try to improve the patients' experiences by improving caregivers' demonstration of courtesy, respect, listening, and clinical explanations. Hospitals have also tried to respect patients by reducing unnecessary ambient noise, streamlining staff communications, reducing patients' wait times, and keeping patients informed about their caregivers as well as their diagnosis, treatment, and discharge information. We need to continually ask ourselves, "What can we as individual physicians do to improve the experience of our patients?" including focusing on improving our ability to provide empathy and support, to answer questions and summarize, and, at times, to simply stop talking so we can listen more.

Communication Training Courses

Today, physicians, at every level of training and practice, can learn and improve communication skills. After several years of planning and researching pilot programs and previous studies, and under the direction of Dr. Adrienne Boissy, the Cleveland Clinic developed the Center for Excellence in Healthcare Communication. The center has various communications training programs designed specifically for all of their doctors, staff, residents, fellows, and students. Thousands of clinicians have received the training. The vast majority of attendees (95%) at their campus courses are Cleveland Clinic caregivers, according to Jennifer Muehle, PMP, Program Coordinator. In an article published in 2016 in the *Journal of General Internal Medicine*, Boissy and her colleagues concluded that their system-wide relationship-centered communication training program improved patient satisfaction scores, physician empathy, and self-efficacy; the training also reduced physician burnout.[2] In other words, better physician communication skills translate into happier patients, more fulfilled physicians, and better organizational environments. Most important, improved communication means a better chance for improved clinical outcomes. Communication skills can and should be part of physicians' continuing education.

Benefits of Physician Communication Training

Improved:
  Clinical outcomes
  Patient satisfaction
  Patient compliance
Decreased:
  Liability
  Costs
  Physician burnout

Source: Cleveland Clinical Center for Excellence in Healthcare Communication.

I have attended, taught, or facilitated several different communication skills training courses throughout my life. In 2018, I had the opportunity to take the communications training course offered by the Cleveland Clinic. The Cleveland Clinic conducts six to eight similar day-long sessions each month, with an average of twelve physician participants in each session taught by two trained physician facilitators. The take-home lesson from this extraordinary program for me was a reinforcement of the foundations of good communications with patients. Specifically, their R.E.D.E. (Relationship, Establishment, Development, and Engagement) program identifies three important stages of the physician–patient relationship during a patient's visit:

> *Phase one: establishment*—this is when we as physicians convey value and respect by welcoming the patient appropriately, collaboratively set an agenda with the patient, and begin to demonstrate empathy
>
> *Phase two: development*—this is when we need to engage in reflective listening, elicit the patient's narrative, and explore the patient's perspective

Phase three: engagement—this is when we share our diagnosis and information, collaboratively develop a treatment plan, provide closure, and remember to encourage a dialogue with the patient throughout the visit.[7]

The full-day program allowed time for practice, feedback, and group collaboration between different types of physicians and trainees. On my day, there was a mix of trainees in internal medicine and orthopedic surgery. The group comradery, sharing, and safe space to practice were all invaluable, as were the lessons on how to encourage patients to express themselves and their concerns early in the patient visit and on how to provide adequate closure.

I asked the medical director Dr. Katie Neuendorf if the Cleveland Clinic would ever make the program available online. She said they had been looking into ways to try to present the program online for the past few years but had not found one that worked. According to Dr. Neuendorf, there seems to be no way to encapsulate the effectiveness of the face-to-face presentation, participation, feedback, and practice sessions of the in-person workshop in an online forum. Perhaps this is really the heart of our learning and practicing human-to-human communication skills. In order to assess ourselves, as well as learn and practice new skills, we need to do it in person and face to face. We cannot use electronic screens, online video, hardware, or software to help us. This may be an area where we need to omit the computer completely—especially when we are trying to improve our human connections with patients and each other.

Today, there are a growing list of medical educational organizations, healthcare plans, and training institutions offering a variety of workshops, single classes, and multiday courses on communication for clinicians. I was in China in 2018 and listened to physicians and hospital employees discuss the need for physician communications programs. It seems the need for discussion and training on this topic is now worldwide. According to the Agency for

Healthcare Research and Quality (AHRQ) at the US Department of Health and Human Services, "the purpose of these programs is to improve providers' effectiveness as both managers of care and educators of patients. It is believed that trained physicians may allocate a greater percent of clinic-visit time to patient education, leading to increased patient knowledge, better compliance with treatment, and improved health outcomes."[8]

Many hospitals and healthcare plans in the United States now offer their own communication training; a few hire outside health communication organizations to run their programs. Some mandate training for all clinicians, and others offer optional courses or provide the instructions as an intervention for physicians with low patient-satisfaction scores or other problems. Communication training programs promise to cover various strategies for improved communication in a relatively short period of time for busy clinicians, often charging $1000 a day or more per practitioner and offering continuing medical education (CME) credits and other incentives. Some of the organizations are listed on the AHRQ website (https://www.ahrq.gov).

Effective communications skills training, whether it is presented as part of a national conference or as an in-house CME course, can offer a supportive environment for clinicians where they can learn specific tools to help communicate with patients, including providing specific interviewing techniques, learning to express compassion, working with time constraints, understanding the patient's perspective, and setting boundaries. Unfortunately, today the obstacles that reduce the quality of our relationship with patients are innumerous: shorter visits, computer screens, electronic health records, unconscious biases, cultural and language differences, misaligned expectations, uncoordinated specialists' consultations, lack of a relationship with the patient, our diminished stature in the patient's eyes, and physicians' own feelings of frustration. According to the AHRQ, "Most practicing physicians have not been taught to appreciate the patient's experience of illness; nor do they learn how to partner with patients and serve as a coach or a guide. As a result, they typically do not know how to communicate with patients in a way that maximizes understanding and involvement in decision-making, lets the patient know that his or her concerns have been heard, and ensures that the care plan meets the needs of the patient."[8]

One of the most obvious obstacles to the patient–physician alliance may be the computer. Dr. Margot Hartunian, a primary care doctor with Beth Israel Deaconess Health Care in Lexington, Massachusetts, uses an ingenious way to integrate the computer into her patient visits. She wheels in her WiFi-connected laptop placed on a small high-topped wooden table into the exam room. With its beautiful wood rounded corners and quiet wheels, Dr. Hartunian maneuvers the small table so it is never between her and her patient. She can stand or sit near it, push it to the side or wheel it in close to the exam table. It never seems obtrusive. Other doctors have hired scribes to take notes so that they can keep their attention and hands free for patient care. Others have tried to come up with alternative solutions using technology including audio recording devices or iPads. But unfortunately, many solutions still interrupt the personal intimacy of the patient–physician human connection in the exam room.

Technology and the electronic universe of the Internet increasingly affect our clinical relationships and interactions in many different ways. Much has been written about the shortcomings of the electronic medical record (EMR), from taking our eyes off the patient in order to type, to cutting and pasting inaccurate information into the patient's chart. But there are many advantages of the EMR. At first, many older physicians rejected EMRs, but some like Dr. Pablo Rodriguez, an obstetrician-gynecologist affiliated with Women and Infants Hospital of Rhode Island, welcomed the EMR and thinks it is a blessing. He practiced for several decades before using the EMR. Today, he says the EMR allows him many "firsts" in his practice, including making his notes more legible and accessible to everyone, always having access to the patient's chart (no more "missing charts"), and having immediate access to seemingly unlimited information and data analysis about each patient. (See Chapter 2 for more discussion about EMR and other technology impacting our healthcare communications.)

While the computer can both intrude and augment our face-to face relationships with patients, it certainly has influenced patients' understanding of their ailments. Patients often search the Internet and consult "Dr. Google" before they arrive in our offices. Sometimes this is advantageous; the patients are more educated and prepared about their symptoms and condition. Sometimes the opposite is true. They may look up symptoms and give themselves an inaccurate diagnose (or more than one) and alarm themselves long before we ever see them. Many patients have a set idea about what they are suffering from and what treatments they want. Some do not want to talk about their symptoms or to be examined. Instead, they just want to request a prescription or a specific test. Some request a referral based on what they have learned from the Internet. In such cases, it may take some additional time and discussion to establish a connection with the patient so that you can make your own assessment and properly take care of them. You might be able to explain how Dr. Google is not always an accurate diagnostician or able to provide a complete therapeutic evaluation of their symptoms and concerns; but often your approach to your clinical interaction may need to be adjusted when the Internet's Dr. Google has already seen the patient. On more than one occasion, after I finish taking a history, examining the patient, and explaining what I think is causing their symptoms, the patient exclaims, "Oh, good that is exactly what I read on the Internet."

Patients may also have read your online patient reviews and expect you to live up (or down) to what other patients have written about you. You may have no established relationship with the patient, whether you are a primary care doctor or a specialist. In this new world of increased expectations, changing roles, lack of physician–patient relationships, and abundance of online medical information, how can we best communicate with patients? Has our job changed in the exam room in the doctoring environment of today? Has our own communication evolved or devolved with the advances (or intrusion) of technology? How can we re-establish and maintain our relationships with our patients in the ever-changing environment of healthcare expectations?

Physician Communication Concerns: What Do Physicians Fear?

There are as many different communication styles as there are physicians. However, many physicians share the same fears and worries when trying to improve their own communication skills with patients. What are physicians most fearful of when it comes to trying to communicate with patients? Here are some common fears physicians express.

1. *"I worry that if I ask my patients too many open-ended questions, they will never stop talking."*

   Once patients start talking, physicians interrupt within several seconds (on average between 18 and 23 seconds).[9] Interestingly, if you let patients talk, without interrupting, they will talk for just about 90 seconds before stopping.[10,11] Patients need to be heard and to tell you everything they are experiencing. They will feel better for having told you everything they came into tell you and for the opportunity to express themselves without being interrupted. As most doctors know, often the diagnosis comes from the history. I often find that patients will give an almost complete history if I just allow them to talk.

2. *"I don't always know how to handle their strong emotions."*

   As physicians, our job is to find solutions to problems and to fix what is broken, injured, or hurting. But according to the Cleveland Clinic and other healthcare communications programs, as physicians, we cannot always "fix" emotions or "mend" all concerns or feelings. What we can do is listen and be present, respectful, and grateful for our patients' ability to share their emotions. We can make sure our patients have been heard, comforted, and supported. We need to identify their emotions accurately and respond to them appropriately. We need to be there for them, encourage them to share with us, witness their predicaments, and offer solace when and where we can.

3. *"I don't have enough time to communicate effectively."*
   It takes less time to communicate effectively with patients than it does to communicate ineffectively. More important, the clinical, professional, and personal benefits of effective and collaborative communications between physicians and patients are numerous.

4. *"Sometimes, there are no tests or treatments needed, there is nothing more I can do for a patient. Then what should I do?"*
   The art of listening can be very therapeutic. Just letting your patients talk and express their emotions can be the most important part of the therapy you offer. Affirming and supporting their feelings and emotions and listening to their fears and opinions is all part of our job as clinicians. Asking them directly about their feelings and expectations and encouraging them to share their concerns should always be part of the discussion.

5. *"Patients don't seem to think I care about them."*
   Being genuine, respectful, and appreciative can be very helpful. Often in medicine, we assume that just by working as a doctor and wearing our white coats, patients should know how much we care for and respect them. They should know we want to understand them and make them feel better. But this is not always communicated by us or understood by our patients. Sometimes we need to use specific words, phrases, questions, and body language to communicate these important messages. We need to ask or say things such as, "Thank you for coming in today," "Thank you for sharing that with me," "What I think I hear you saying is . . . ," and "What were you hoping for during today's visit with me?"

6. *"I worry that becoming an 'excellent communicator' means agreeing with everything the patient wants."*

A healthy relationship between physician and patient does not mean agreeing with everything the patients says or requests. A healthy relationship with a patient does not mean "agreement on everything, unlimited time, tolerance of boundary violations or practicing outside your usual scope of practice," according to the Cleveland Clinic's Center for Excellence in Healthcare Communication. It does mean, according to the center, "making an emotional connection, showing mutual respect and genuine interest in the patient perspective and psychosocial context and a shared commitment to a positive outcome." In all relationships, we need to learn how to agree to disagree. We need to value ourselves and our opinions just as we do our patients and their opinions, while acknowledging that the stressful environment of healthcare and the uncertainty and emotions of illness can strain any interaction.

What Do Patients Want? What Do Physicians Want?

Patients and physicians want the same thing: to be respected, to be heard, to have a therapeutic interaction, and to have an improved outcome for the patient. When it comes down to it, our job is to listen, and their job is to talk. But we need to provide patients with the right questions, information, environment, support, and time so that they will be encouraged to talk. We need to answer the patients' questions and give them honest explanations that will help them. Patients do not want to be rushed and treated like multiple-choice questions, "Aha, I know what you have, the answer is B!" Patients also do not want to hear a medical lecture or public health speech from us. They want a dialogue with us, not a monologue from us. Having a therapeutic interaction takes time to listen and time to be present. It also takes patience and compassion. Knowing that we have the same goals as the patient of an accurate diagnosis and an improved outcome is central to connecting and communicating. Unfortunately, without an established relationship, patients do not know who we are or how much we care. We often don't understand their background, their lives, or their experiences. They don't think we have the time or interest in hearing all of their concerns or questions. And it seems that both patients and physicians are strapped for time.

A Harris poll conducted in 2015 indicated that three out of five adults would choose telehealth visits to replace in-person visits for things such as follow-up visits, eye infections, skin checks, and minor ailments if this option were offered by doctors, according to an article published in *Business Wire*.[12] What does this say about the patients' comfort and satisfaction with face-to-face communications with their doctors? What does this say about the way some would prefer to have their healthcare delivered? If patients prefer efficiency over an in-person visit, or if they prefer to search their symptoms online instead of seeking advice from us, then the nature of our relationship is surely changing. It seems that computer screens, in some instances, may have replaced our listening ears and our healing hands. However, while patients can search the Internet, "Dr. Google" cannot make a diagnosis, provide empathy, or care for them like we can. But access to online health information and a lack of a personal relationships with patients have possibly increased the miscommunication and misaligned expectations between us. As physicians, we have to remember that our job is to be reflective and empathic listeners, accurate diagnosticians, and excellent caregivers. We also need to remember to let the patients tell their story, including what information they believe to be true about their symptoms. Here is an essay I wrote a few years ago about how I learned this lesson.

Let Them Tell Their Story

In 1984, researchers Beckman and Frankel found that on average doctors allow patients to talk for just several seconds before interrupting.* Subsequent studies confirmed this finding, and much has been written about the impact on not only how it makes the patient feel but how it actually limits the clinical information physicians are able to learn from patients. But today more than three decades later, even several seconds may seem like an eternity in our instant electronic age. I worry that we are not only still interrupting patients but also barely allowing them to speak.

As an internist I sometimes work in the fast-paced environment of a hospital walk-in clinic. On a typical day, the triage nurse initially interviews the patients and documents their problems: the productive cough, the stomachache, the painful swollen knee, or the hot enlarging abscess and fever since the trip to South America. Before I walk in the exam room, I read the nurse's note including the patient's chief complaint, history of present illness, vital signs, medications, allergies, and past medical history.

During my first few years as a doctor, I would knock on the exam room door, rush in to introduce myself and then almost all in one breath would say, "So I understand you have been coughing up green sputum for a week and have a fever. You have not traveled in the past year. You don't have muscle aches, asthma, or a smoking history. You've had your flu shot. Have you had any wheezing or shortness of breath?"

Despite my enthusiasm and earnest, detailed approach, some patients would look somewhat confused and disappointed. I was often taken aback at their lack of appreciation for my thorough questioning and services as a doctor. Yes, in medical school I had learned how to take a full history from a patient in a relaxed setting, but the reality of the number of patients to be seen combined with the need to quickly collect data sometimes pushed me (and my physician peers) to assume a frenzied attempt at history gathering instead of a calm interaction and dialogue with patients.

I learned relatively quickly that patients need to talk, and I needed to listen. As humans, we need to tell our story—especially when we are sick. And we need someone, especially the doctor, to listen. By not asking open-ended questions such as, "How can I help you?" or "What brings you hear today?" or providing the right prompts such as, "Tell me what is going on," patients do not feel cared for, and we miss hearing important details in their full story.

People living in various cultures, from ancient to modern day, from Native Americans to Tahitians, from Africans to Irish, use storytelling to reflect and reconnect. Today, the spoken word compiled into a personal narrative is how we still communicate and connect. It is how we understand each other's worlds. Neuroscientists have documented the neural connections between the brains of one person telling a story and another person listening.† The activity in each brain becomes aligned during the conversation; it seems our brains are wired for storytelling. And there is no more important time to do this than when we are not feeling well.

Patients need to explain what's going on and describe what is troubling them in their own narrative. They need to elucidate the details, timeline, and understanding of their illness. We, as doctors, need to allow the patients to stammer at the difficult parts, shed a tear at the sadness, wince at the pain, and pause when they are lost. This narrative pathway between a sharing patient and a listening, caring doctor is paramount for good communication and good care.

Speaking and listening are intimate exchanges. Our voices are unique creations that begin with a breath of molecules deep inside of us. When we speak and someone listens, the sound waves enter the body of the listener and alter thoughts, feelings, and perceptions. To have your voice heard or to listen to another's voice is a deep, personal, and profound experience. It can also be comforting and healing.

Like many newly minted doctors, I was simply firing a string of closed-ended questions at patients after a brief recap of the information in their chart. I was soliciting clinical details so that I could make an accurate diagnosis and give them the right treatment plan quickly.

Do you have a headache? No.

Sore throat? No.

Previous problems with that knee? Yes.

Any blood in your diarrhea? No.

Some closed-ended questions are okay (and certainly clinically important), but the first several questions of the conversation you have with patients need to be open ended. Without asking any open-ended questions, I had effectively muzzled my patients from telling their story of illness. I was asking for relevant data, but unfortunately, I had stolen their individual narratives from them.

I was not giving them the opportunity to describe their symptoms, concerns, and emotions in their own vocabulary. I was depriving myself from hearing their accounts. Our communication was incomplete, mechanical, and one-sided. I was conducting an interview that may have sounded more like a cross-examination or inquisition—not a human conversation. The personal exchange of a deeper human connection was lost.

The patients were frustrated, and so was I.

Today, I use a different approach.

"How are you? What is going on?" I ask. And then I listen. Really listen.

It may sound simple. It is.

It may sound simplistic. It is not.

And no, we don't have long periods of time together. But however long we do have, I know I have to allow them enough time to convey their experience. Most important, I let them talk first. I let them finish their sentences and tell me their full stories so that I can learn about them—and their stories.

How I introduce myself, shake their hand, and ask those first few questions sets the tone of the entire visit. These moments are critical. I convey a message of caring by listening. The patients experience comfort by sharing. Patients usually tell a complete history if you allow them to. Unfortunately, in our current world of instant-data-texting-pop-up-electronic-record-data-collection-patient visits, we may have forgotten how to slow down and prompt patients' vocal histories.

We might benefit by remembering how attentive we are to a friend describing a visit to the Grand Canyon or the birth of their child or the death of an elderly parent. We let them tell us about the experience. We do not sum up their story and then shoot off a series of yes or no questions. We listen with anticipation, interest, and kindness. We must do the same with our patients.

We must be a witness to their personal chronicle.

That is what a doctor does. That is what a hurt or sick patient wants us to do. That is effective communication between patient and clinician.

As the renowned physician Sir William Osler said, "Listen to your patient. He [or she] is telling you the diagnosis."

They are telling us their story. And we must listen.

Storytelling preceded the written word. While the printing press diminished our reliance on oral stories, let us not allow electronic medical records to diminish our reliance on patients' stories—or our willingness to listen to them.

* H. B. Beckman and R. M. Frankel, "The Effect of Physician Behavior on the Collection of Data," *Ann Intern Med.*,1984;101;692–696.

† L. Silbert, C. Honey, E. Simony, D. Poeppel, and U. Hasson, "Coupled Neural Systems Underlie the Production and Comprehension of Naturalistic Narrative Speech," *Proc Natl Acad Sci USA*, 2014;111(43):E4687–E4696.

Shared Silence—Embrace the Pause

To sit in silence with other people is one of the most intimate experiences imaginable.

—Doug Toft[13]

In a clinical setting, silence or a pause can represent many different emotions from our patients, such as fear, exasperation, exhaustion, shock, awe, anger, concern, sadness, or confusion, to name just a few. But sitting in silence with our patients for a few seconds or a few minutes can be very therapeutic, for them and for us.

Why do we feel like we need to fill every minute with chatter, questions, or explanations? It is okay to embrace the pause, exhale, and give the patient and yourself a break. Our verbal exchanges can be like a dance with an escalating pace and volume at times. What if we just took a moment and sat with some of our patients as we would a friend near a stream? What if we allowed ourselves to share a moment of silence with our patients? What if we were not afraid to just be quiet with our patients?

Silences occur naturally in all conversations, if we allow them. They can help recalibrate the rhythm between you and your patient. You may have been rushing for the last several hours in your busy day while your patient may have been sitting in silence waiting for you. Having the same emotional rhythm or pace between you and the patient is very important. Silence can allow you to observe the mood of your patient and feel the tenor of the room. Silence may occur spontaneously or may emerge in response to a strong emotional moment. Sometimes after a patient says something very powerful, perhaps about the recent loss of their spouse or the fear of a diagnosis, I say, "I am so very sorry" or, "I hear what you are saying and it sounds like you are sad, concerned, or fearful." I then try to stop and just embrace the pause—allow the simple act of sitting in silence and observing the two of us together to comfort and soothe the patient.

> I often regret that I have spoken; never that I have been silent.
> —Publilius Syrus

Sometimes we avoid silence because it feels awkward. Our lives our generally filled with noise, and our days are busy with sound and activity. The time we are with patients, we need to gather information, ask them questions, and encourage them to explain in detail what is wrong. But a few appropriate pauses or natural moments of silence can actually improve our time with patients in three ways. First, silence can slow down the pace of the room. Often, you will hear people exhale during a pause. Second, allowing some silence can show how comfortable you are in the room and with the patient. Third, it gives the patient an opportunity to say something spontaneous and not just give another answer in response to your questions.

> We are embraced by silence and silence cares for us deeply. In the embrace of silence we sense the essence of living things radiating loudly.
> —Robert Rabbin

A few moments of shared silence with your patient may be worth an hour of noisy verbal exchange. Do not deprive yourself or your patients the comfort and intimacy of silence when it naturally occurs. You will save energy and time; you will gain a calm connection with your patient. You may observe, hear, or intuit important clinical information from the quiet time you spend in their presence.

Specific Goals of Communicating
with Patients

Of course, our ultimate goal is to help the patient achieve optimal health status. We know that the better we are at communicating, the better chance we have of achieving that goal. If Aristotle (384–322 BC), the Greek philosopher and scientist, could accompany us while we are taking care of patients today, he might remind us of what he thought of as the critical components of good communication: ethos, pathos, and logos (Figure 1.1). Ethos is our credibility or character, pathos is our emotional or personal connection with the patient, and logos is the logic we are using and the actual words we are saying. Our rhetoric, he wrote, is "worthy of systematic and scientific study."[14]

The patient's perception of us and our communication skills rests on what Aristotle described as this "rhetorical triangle." The image illustrates how the three components are dependent on each other, ultimately define how our patients perceive us, and perhaps ultimately determine our ability to achieve our clinical goals. If we use an abrupt or off-putting tone or style, the patient may think we are not credible or trustworthy (ethos), and the communication

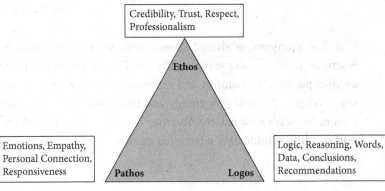

Figure 1.1 Aristotle's rhetorical triangle.

triangle collapses. If we are rushed, brief, or dismissive, we may not make an emotional connection with the patient (pathos). If we use reasoning, with data and words that are not understandable or logical (logos) for the patient, then our connection with the patient is interrupted. The patient will be confused by the information we are providing and not appreciate our intentions.

Establishing an emotional connection with a patient always requires respect, time, and patience. I enter with a warm hello and open-ended questions and then try to assess the situation before we begin, dipping a toe in before we enter the pool of true interaction. I cannot assume anything about the patients' history, mood, or expectations until I spend time with them. I must be aware and cautious of first impressions and my own biases.

Of course, preparation is key. I need to learn as much as I can from the medical record, my own notes, the nurse, or any other source to help me determine the best approach to take with the patient before walking into the room. After many years, I have learned to trust what my nurses say about the patients' mood and interactions that occurred before I see them. But I also try to imagine a "clean slate" when I walk in the room. I don't make any assumptions. I try to stay open and enter calmly, with a smile and a welcome gesture. I do not assume I am going to get a warm reception or that I can predict how the patient will interact with me. I need to get to know my patients, their expectations, and their fears by asking them the right questions and letting them talk. I need to listen and observe as much as I can. I want to make an emotional or human connection. They need to know that I care.

Small gestures can be important. I try to watch my volume and pacing so that I am not shouting or speaking too quickly. I want to make sure my verbal and nonverbal language is open, welcoming, and caring and appropriate for the patient. I need to match the tenor of my approach and interaction to each individual patient and circumstance. I want to try to have a therapeutic interaction with each patient.

Important Lessons of Communication with Patients

- Greet patients with a smile and a handshake or other respectful gesture.
- Sit down and make eye contact.
- Have a dialogue with the patient—not a monologue.
- Do not interrupt.
- Listen, reflect back what they are saying (reflective listening).
- Allow for pauses and silence.
- Provide a plan and closure at the end of the visit.
- Make sure the patient understands.
- Make sure the patient has no more questions.

Source: The Cleveland Clinic.[7]

Aristotle and modern-day communication experts encourage us to articulate our specific goals before any encounter with a patient. If we can define our specific goals beforehand, then our mission will be clear as to why we want to be good communicators with each patient in the first place. Remember each day why you are seeing patients. What are your goals and what is your mission with each patient?

Goals of Communicating with Patients

1. To gather information
2. To listen to the patient's needs and concerns
3. To offer empathy and support
4. To assess their expectations
5. To encourage questions
6. To explain your clinical thinking, diagnosis, and treatment
7. To make a connection
8. To foster a therapeutic relationship

Physician attitudes that can lead to poor communication include emotional burnout, insecurity, intolerance of diagnostic uncertainty, and negative bias toward specific health conditions.[15] Inadequate training in psychosocial medicine and a limited knowledge of the patient's health condition can lead to difficult encounters.[15] If we are anxious, depressed, exhausted, overworked, dealing with personal health issues or situational stressors or sleep deprivation, our patients will suffer; and if we have difficulty feeling and expressing empathy or are easily frustrated, we will not be good doctors.[15]

Learning from Other Communication Training

Can we learn from other types of communication training? During advanced cardiovascular life support (ACLS) training, communication is emphasized as the most important component needed in an emergency situation. The six essentials for communicating during an emergency are respect, constructive criticism, constructive intervention, closed-loop communications, algorithms, and a team leader.[16,17]

While many physicians do not work in emergency situations requiring the level of communication to run a code, all of us work in unpredictable, stressful, emotional, and sometimes chaotic environments with individuals who we do not always fully know. We can learn from the underlying principles of the ACLS training in our communication with patients and peers in any type of situation if we respect others, make sure our communications are clear and understood, make sure we fully understand what the other person is saying, and are willing to question, converse, and relate with reverence.

In any communications training, including "organizational or institutional communications" or even "self-help and communication for couples" or other similar courses, attendees learn about themselves as well as interpersonal skills to develop understanding and empathy for each other, specific methods for effective communication, nurturing, influencing, and resolving and repairing relationship conflict. Of course, "self-help for couples" communication skills may not seem appropriate for the physician–patient relationship, but there are many aspects of the training we might consider with our patients and our peers, including the type of respect and caring needed in any human relationship. While "love may mean never saying you are sorry," in medicine we certainly can say "I'm sorry" with our patients and our peers. "I am sorry I am running late," "I am sorry I forgot to call you," "I am sorry to tell you that you have pneumonia," or "I am sorry you have been waiting so long to see me." Gratitude is also very important. "Thank you for telling me that," and "Thank you for coming in today." Respect + gratitude + empathy = care.

Relationship Skills Building

1. **Show caring and warmth.** There are so many nonphysical ways of showing warmth, from a smile to shared silence. Physical affection is not appropriate, of course, for a physician–patient relationship, and individuals react differently to different physical gestures from hugs to touching a shoulder or a hand. But we can certainly show kindness and caring by small and large gestures, from shaking hands to helping patients on and off the table. One person described how touched she was when a doctor who was caring for her dying husband helped carry his shoes from one room to the next. Showing warmth toward a patient can come in a variety of nonphysical and professionally appropriate physical ways.

2. **Be patient with each patient.** If we are rushed or abrupt with patients, they are not going to feel cared for. If we cannot

patiently listen, they will not feel we care. Just like with other relationships, we need to sit down and give them the time they need. Learning to make the most of the time you have and giving the patient your undivided attention for that time is key. Learning to listen and to accept your patients' unique qualities and never losing your curiosity about your patients or their lives are important. Learn how you can show respect to your patients, and you will learn more about them and how you can help them.

3. **Listen carefully and thoughtfully.** Be a good listener by leaning in, nodding, responding with "yes" or "uh-huh," and looking directly into your patients' eyes. Note not only the emotions of their words but also the cues of their body language.

4. **Be thoughtful with small and large acts.** Small acts can show you care. You can certainly show thoughtfulness by remembering important personal information about a patient's family. You can also pick up something they have dropped or ask them if they need a glass of water. Comment on the book they are reading or ask them what they are knitting. These interactions also give you a minute to put down your stethoscope and just relate human to human. Large acts of thoughtfulness mean going the extra mile in every aspect of their care. Take care of them as if they were a family member.

5. **Show gratitude.** Showing appreciation shows respect for the patients and their time. Thank patients for their questions. Thank them for sharing information with you. Thank them for coming into to see you and being on time.

6. **Be calm, gentle, and understanding.** A calm, gentle, and understanding approach with most patients is much more beneficial than the opposite approach. Each patient is different.

Each set of circumstances is different. We should remain gentle, open, humble, and understanding.

7. **Be open to their questions and ideas.** Patients have their own concerns and ideas about their symptoms. They have their own ideas about the diagnosis and appropriate treatment. We need to elicit their thoughts, reasoning, and fears. We may know more about medicine, but they know more about their bodies, emotions, and lives than we do. Never assume you know everything about the patient or their symptoms, concerns, feelings, and lives.

8. **Learn to agree to disagree.** We are not going to agree on everything. We need to set personal and professional boundaries. We can always listen and respond with respect. Losing control and becoming emotional rarely help solve any problems. Recognize when you are stressed and need to take a time-out. On more than one occasion, I have asked a patient to excuse me for a minute. I then just step outside the room for a few minutes. The patient may think I am answering a page or answering a question from my nurse, but in all honesty, I am just taking a few minutes to breathe and calm myself. Once I step back into the room, I am always amazed at how an emotionally charged situation will diffuse by just taking a break for a few minutes. Generally, I re-enter the room, the heightened emotions have resolved, and the conversation proceeds smoothly.

Learning from Other Professions

How do other professions connect and communicate with people? Professionals, including journalists, clergy, teachers, and actors, must relate and develop relationships with their readers, their congregation, their students, and their audiences. They have many of the same concerns and face many of the same barriers and difficulties as physicians when trying to connect and communicate with others. We may be able to learn something from each of them.

Journalists

Journalists interview a variety of people in a variety of difficult situations. Award winning news producer and video documentarian Wonbo Woo has worked for network television shows, including ABC 20/20 and NBC Nightly News. In the course of his career, he has interviewed thousands of people, from soldiers in war-torn areas and survivors of national tragedies to the parents of a transgender child and clergy who have lost their faith. He not only asks people to share their personal information but also asks them to do it in front of a camera. I asked him to share his secrets on how he is able to make deep and sometimes quick connections with people in difficult situations and encourage them to share information with him—information he needs in order to tell an important news story. Here are his keys to good communication and a successful interview. As one of my medical students said, "he could be talking to physicians with this advice."

Person-to-Person Communication Advice from a Journalist

- Know what information you need to get before the interview.
- Prepare beforehand.
- Read as much as you can.
- Understand their story before going in.
- Go in prepared to listen.
- Listen to the emotional cues in their voices.
- Watch the physical cues in their body language.
- Listen between the lines.
- Respect them at all times.
- Make sure you have eye-to-eye contact.
- Treat them as humans.
- Manage the stress (yours and theirs).
- Ask them about their concerns.
- Try to connect in that moment.
- Be there in that moment (cut everything else out).

Like many successful journalists, Wonbo loves meeting new people, and he loves hearing people's stories. We should feel the same about our patients. We should never lose our curiosity about our patients and our interest in their lives.

Clergy

Several years ago, ministers, priests, rabbis, and other clergy made regular visits to see many patients in the hospital. At most hospitals, they would check in at the front desk and would be given a list of the patients who identified as Catholic, Christian, Jewish, Muslim, or other religion. Members of the clergy would then take the list and walk the halls of the hospitals finding these patients and visiting with them. The patients may or may not have been members of their congregations or synagogues, but clergy were allowed open access to these patients to provide them with spiritual care while they were hospitalized. Today, while individual patients or their family members may request their priest or rabbi visit them in the hospital, many of the routine spiritual rounds and other regular types of clergy visits have greatly diminished or gone away completely at some hospitals. There are a variety of reasons for this, including that patients spend less time in the hospitals than they used to so that by the time the rabbi or the minister hears about the patients in the hospital, they may be discharged. Also, there are more rules and regulations concerning patients' private information, including their religious preferences, and some clergy feel intimidated or unwelcome by some hospital settings today. I sat down with Rebecca Spencer, Senior Minister at Central Congregational Church in Providence, Rhode Island, who used to spend many hours a week doing these visits and, like many, misses them. While there are certainly still clergy present in hospitals, the declining number of regular hospital visits seems to be a reflection of many changes in our healthcare environment.

I asked Reverend Spencer about the art of listening and talking to members of her congregation in and out of the hospital. She stressed that people overwhelmingly just need to be listened to. But listening takes time and presence. Spencer calls it the "ministry of presence." I think the problem for physicians is that although are we worried that we don't have the time to listen, we are not always emotionally present for the time we are with patients. Worse yet, if we are on "auto-pilot," for example, thinking that it is a straightforward case of another upper respiratory infection or urinary tract infection and we don't need to be fully emotionally present, then we and our patients will miss out on the therapeutic human connection of presence. Another problem for physicians is that we are often much more interested in the objective data than the subjective data. Patients want to share both with us. They want to tell us what their high fever felt like or how the itch kept them awake all night, along with their other worries, fears, and expectations.

Time is a commodity we all seem to have less and less of. Other professions, including members of the clergy and journalists, seem to have less time, too. But some individuals seem to help manage this obstacle by being more present. Journalist Wonbo Woo says he relies on "being present in the moment." He says that no matter how little time he has with the people he is interviewing, he tries not to be distracted and keeps his total focus on the other person and what they are saying. Rebecca Spencer's "ministry of presence" means she is fully there for her congregates when she is sitting with them. Perhaps we as physicians need to think about this as well. We must be fully emotionally, physically, and intellectually present for our patients every minute we have with them. We cannot be thinking about the next patient, or the last patient, or a lab or x-ray result we are waiting for. For a few minutes, we need to just sit and listen. Reverend Spencer also believes it is important for clergy (and physicians) to ask people what they need and what we can do to help. When was the last time you walked into a patient's room and simply asked, "How can I help?" and then with laser-like focus really listened and observed?

Rabbi Leslie Y. Gutterman of Temple Beth-El in Providence, Rhode Island feels strongly about listening to each other. He wrote the following in the Providence Journal on December 8, 2018:

> [I]t cannot be overstated that listening in an openhearted, attentive manner may be more helpful than we might imagine. Absorbing someone's anguish by the unspoken reassurance of our presence can mean a lot. Therefore, the best wisdom is often: Don't do something, just stand there!
>   —Rabbi Leslie Y. Gutterman

Rabbi Gutterman's personal experience with doctors has led him to believe it is important for doctors to learn about their patients no matter how much or how little time they have together. Years ago, when his first wife was diagnosed with leukemia and just a year before she died, they had an experience with a physician who was abrupt and abrasive. Rabbi Gutterman felt that the physician had prepared a speech for him and his wife and never took the time to get to know them or to listen to their concerns or questions. He learned in that painful moment that physicians who cannot stop to listen and learn about their patients do not seem like physicians who care.

Person-to-Person Communications Advice from Clergy

- Listen to the patient.
- Be fully present when you are with the patient.
- Answer the patient's questions.
- Ask the patient, "Is there anything we did not talk about today?"
- Let the patient know you will stay in touch and you won't abandon him or her.
- Ask the patient, "What did you hear me say?"
- Always ask, "Is there anything else?"

Educators

Educator Cotty Saltonstall taught school for forty-six years at Dexter (Dexter Southfield) School in Brookline, Massachusetts. Now retired, his advice about relating to his students can certainly be helpful to physicians trying to relate and interact with their patients. Finding a common ground, for example, asking patients about their children at college or how their garden is this year, is as important as the first handshake of greeting or the exchange of smiles after the closure of the visit and, similar to communicating with students, may make the difference in how well you connect with them.

The art of relating to children—and others—derives, I believe, from listening to them as opposed to talking at them. When students realize that one is truly interested in hearing what they have to say, be it about weekend activities, favorite foods, games, sports, books, or anything they might like to talk about, the foundation of a relationship is formed. As time passes, trust is usually built, resulting in a strengthening of the connection between teacher and pupil, and as that evolves, it becomes easier to inspire those whom one is trying to teach. Throughout the process, the teacher is able to recognize areas of strength and weakness, and address them, helping the child to gain in confidence and start to dare to tackle new challenges.

In summary, although I retired some years ago, I believe that much of what I learned about relating to and inspiring children still holds true today and also applies to others in other professions. For those adults who are willing to listen to those whom they are mentoring, teaching, guiding, or treating, the rewards are many."

—Cotty Saltonstall

Actors

I asked a professional theater actor, Fred Sullivan Jr., how actors "show" empathy. He quickly educated me on the fact that actors don't "show" anything—they embody a character who is feeling an emotion such as empathy. In learning a character, they ask themselves, "What if what was happening on stage to my character was happening to me?" and then they feel the emotions of their character. Of course, as physicians we can learn the verbal language and nonverbal techniques of showing empathy, but unless we really feel it for our patients and their stories, no one will believe us. We must always ask ourselves, "What if that was me or my mother or my grandfather or my son on the table?"

The take-home lesson for me in talking to a professional theater actor was to remember that as physicians we need to think more about how we feel and embody the virtues of medicine, including kindness, patience, humility, and respect, and then practice them— not try to emulate some technique that we think our patients will perceive as empathic or respectful. We must be empathic and respectful. We must listen and relate. We must care both about and for our patients.

The Words We Use

Like many professions, medicine has its own language. Many of the words sound scientific, obtuse, or archaic. Most have Latin origins. Some have English or Germanic or just odd pronunciations. During our training, these words seems to invite us into the secret society of medicine. The jargon is part of our "in-doctor-ination" or induction. Why do we say "palpate" when we could say "touch?" Why do we say "hydrate" when we mean "drink?" "Inhale" instead of breathe? "Expire" instead of "die?" Why do we use so many military metaphors such as "doctor's orders" or "war on cancer" or "armamentarium against cancer?" Interestingly enough, the first definition of armamentarium in the *Oxford English Living Dictionary* is not about war but about medicine. It reads, "the medicines, equipment, and techniques available to a medical practitioner," with the example "leeches of the medieval armamentarium are making a comeback in modern medicine."

Using jargon puts us at a distance from patients. It separates the landscape of human connection, understanding, and emotion. Do the words of our profession keep us from feeling our emotions and separate us from our patients? Do they place an artificial and imposing barrier between us? Are they harming our ability to communicate and connect with patients?

When University of Rhode Island Professor of English and creative nonfiction author Mary Cappello spoke to my medical students at Alpert Medical School at Brown University, she challenged them to think of synonyms we use in our everyday language and in medicine that appear very close in meaning but in fact may have nuanced or not so nuanced distinctions. Words like "listen and hear"; "cut and incise"; "care and concern"; and "learn and know." Professor Cappello then gave us a list of five medical terms she wanted us to think about: documenting; observing; witnessing; attending; and studying.

Each of these words carries a different meaning for physicians in relation to patients and for writers in relation to their subjects. What this lesson exposed and illustrated was the distance from the subject (the patient) we feel (or don't feel) by using certain clinical words. It also raised the question, is the patient the subject or the object in our sentences? We quickly realized that we rarely ask ourselves what our words and our sentence structure really mean to us and to our patients. Most words in medicine may place us further from the patient, not closer. Perhaps we need to think more about the specific words we use with patients and among ourselves and how they make us act and feel.

Patients know we have these unique and specialized words in our profession. Sometimes they use medical jargon in front of us to try to get closer or to show us that they may, too, be in the secret society of medicine. When a patient says something to me in medical-ese such as "Is my PO$_2$ coming up?" or "Did my x-ray show a one-centimeter calcified lung nodule in the left upper lobe?" I often ask if they work in medicine. Sometimes they do, and sometimes they do not. If they work in medicine as a clinician, our conversation is often then filled with medical terms and often becomes less emotionally connected. This is not for the better. We need to be aware of the words we use with all of our patients and try to avoid technical jargon to keep the caring human connection established. The words we use not only set us apart as a profession but also may make the patient feel like an object in a scientific experiment. Capello asks us specifically of how we thought of the patient—and how our language reveals the answer. Is the patient doing something or having something done to them? Are their stories and experiences and emotions being validated? Are ours? Are we performing the action or are we removed from the action of palpating or cutting or repairing? Are we partners or parents or paternalistic caregivers? Listen to and note the words you use. How do these words confuse, alienate, and objectify—or reassure, calm, and help us care for our patients and ourselves as physicians?

The words we use in front of patients carry great power and influence. We need to be thoughtful and judicious in the selection of the specific words we speak when caring for patients. Lest you think our words do not matter, think of the three words that begin some of the most important and pivotal sentences, "The doctor said. . . ." Whether we are talking with patients about important recommendations to stop smoking, lose weight, or use condoms or we are explaining a serious diagnosis or describing a therapy, our exact word selection matters.

Our words can comfort, educate, and heal. But unfortunately, they can also hurt, insult, or judge. We need to be careful not to retraumatize those who have experienced trauma, we need to be respectful about the use of pronouns for the transgender community, and for all patients of all ages, ethnicities, and socioeconomic and educational levels. We need to use words that are clear, unbiased, helpful, and healing regardless of whether our patients look like we do or not.

Once I was seeing a young man about a rash on his legs. After describing the history of the rash, I examined him. He was a pleasant young professional man who had been bothered by the rash for several weeks. In the middle of the visit, he looked up at me squarely and politely and said, "Doctor, you know that I was born as a woman right?" His transgender status had nothing to do with his rash. And because I had recently written an article about transgender care and moderated a panel for medical students about caring for transgender patients, I knew to say, "Yes, but you identify as a man, right?" He smiled and nodded. I continued to refer to him as a man for the rest of the visit. I was so thankful I knew the right words to say to support him and care for him. We need to be aware of the specific words, including pronouns, nouns, verbs, adjectives, and adverbs, that we use with every patient.

Nonverbal Communication: Our Body Language

Just as careful listening is critical to understanding our verbal pronouncements, so careful observation is vital to comprehending our body language.

—Joe Navarro, FBI agent and author of *What Every Body is Saying*

The body never lies.

—Martha Graham

Most physicians receive little or no training about reading body language—that of their patients or their own. This is unfortunate because an estimated 60 to 65% of interpersonal communication is conveyed through nonverbal behaviors.[18] And while most nonverbal behaviors are unconscious, they may represent a more accurate depiction of what the patient is thinking or feeling.[19]

For the most part, we observe body language subconsciously. Learning how to consciously observe, note, and assess the meaning of various physical gestures, postures, and movements can help you better understand your patients. There is a reason that law enforcement and other professions use body language to help in assessment and communication. Think about some of the body language you observe (or express) on a daily basis with patients. Think about the body language you should be observing in the exam room and elsewhere in your environment.

Positive Body Language in the Exam Room

- How did you greet the patient (handshake or other gesture)?
- Are you sitting at eye level with the patient?
- Have you removed any physical obstacles (computer or desk) between you and the patient?
- Are your facial expressions warm and comforting?
- Are you leaning forward?
- Are your arms and legs uncrossed?
- Are you mirroring the patient's body language and expressions (isopraxism)?
- Are you physically respectful and appropriately comforting during history taking and physical exam?

Negative Body Language in the Exam Room

- Are you standing?
- Are your toes pointing toward the door?
- Are your arms or legs crossed?
- Are you leaning away?

- Are your hands in your pockets or behind your back?
- Are you looking uninterested or angry?
- Is your hand on the door knob?
- Are you glancing at the clock or the door?
- Are you checking your smart phone?
- Are your hands or eyes on a computer?
- Are you looking harried, hurried, or inpatient?

Your Patient's Body Language

- What is the patient doing when you walk in?
- How is the patient's posture?
- Is the patient standing, sitting, or lying down when talking to you?
- Is the patient straining to look up at you?
- What is the patient's facial expressions saying to you?
- Is the patient avoiding making eye contact with you?
- What are the patient's hands and feet doing while the patient is talking to you?
- Are the patient's arms or legs crossed or feet twitching?
- Are the patient's physical gestures or posture inconsistent with the patient's verbal message?

Here are a few specific tips:

1. **Eyes.** Making eye contact is very important in communication. If someone doesn't make eye contact, it can mean that person is angry, hurt, bored, disinterested, or even lying. It can also indicate nervousness or a submissive nature. Blinking rate can speed up when people are stressed but also when they are lying, especially if they touch their mouth or eyes at the same time. Looking up and to the right can indicate a lie. Looking up and to the left can occur when a person is trying to recall an actual memory.

2. **Feet.** Although many people think hands or eyes are the most emotionally revealing aspects of our bodies, experts say it is actually our feet. Next time you are with a patient, take a look at the patient's feet (and at your own). Are they fidgeting? Tapping? Crossed at the ankles? Pointing toward the door? They may be telling you something different than the words being spoken.

3. **Hands.** One common gesture we may see in patients is clasping or squeezing hands together. This indicates fear or discomfort. Clasped hands with interwoven fingers can mean anxiety and frustration. Hiding one's hands or putting them in one's pockets can indicate mistrust or reluctance. If you notice patients' hands in their pockets, they may not trust you or be interested in what you have to say. (They may also just be cold.)

4. **Crossed arms or legs.** If your patient is exhibiting a defensive posture, something is wrong. You may want to take a break, move on, or ask some open-ended questions about how the patient is feeling because he or she is clearly self-protecting or indicating a closed posture. If the patient's legs or arms are crossed, try to find out what is going on.

The skills you have developed throughout your life when it comes to reading another person's nonverbal cues will likely be what you use in the clinic and your career. But like all aspects of our communication, increasing your awareness about the nonverbal communication between you and your patient and improving your skills in this area can improve your understanding of each other—and may help you provide better care.

Teaching Communication Skills to Trainees

I think we learn most about the types of doctors we'll become from watching our preceptors and residents and learning from

them if they do something particularly well or not so well from
our vantage point.

—Medical student

During clinical training, students witness both positive and negative
examples of communication styles in their attendings and senior
residents. In other words, they are learning by watching us. They
certainly can learn from different types of examples and can decide
which behaviors to emulate and which to reject. Although we hope
they have many more good examples to emulate, unfortunately
many attendings who have been in practice longer than fifteen years
may have never had formal communication skills training. It is
only over the past decade or so that medical schools and residency
training programs have instituted regular standardized communication skills into the curriculum. Practicing physicians may have few
opportunities for communications training once they are busy in
practice, and unless the training is mandated, few may actually sign
up. While many attendings may be excellent communicators with
their patients and staff, others are not. The truth is, most practicing
physicians need to improve their communication skills, and there is
a great necessity for formal institutional training in this area.

I am still learning how to balance wanting to get to know a person,
versus needing the necessary info to help manage their condition.

—Medical student

I want to hear their whole life story [but] then I remember it's
only a 15-minute appointment.

—Medical student

The Accreditation Council for Graduate Medical Education
(ACGME) identifies communication and interpersonal skills (CIS)
as one of the six core competencies for residents to learn along

with patient care, medical knowledge, practice-based learning and improvement, professionalism, and system-based practice. And through various courses throughout medical school and examinations such as the Objective Structured Clinical Exam (OSCE) and the US Medical Licensing Examination (USMLE) Step 2 Clinical Skills Exam, we try to teach trainees to effectively exchange information, to be active listeners and articulate speakers, and to develop meaningful relationships. But once trainees begin seeing patients, why do they learn so much by simply observing?

Observational learning most often occurs when a person lacks confidence in his or her own knowledge or abilities; when the situation is confusing, ambiguous, or unfamiliar; or when there is an authoritative person present, according to renowned social psychologist Albert Bandura at Stanford University. I cannot think of a better description than that of young trainees beginning their clinical training. We need to remember that when residents and students are following us, our communication skills are even more important because they are observing and learning from us. Ultimately, the hidden curriculum for our trainees is the way we conduct ourselves and demonstrate human connection with our patients, family members, colleagues, and staff—and, of course, how we communicate directly with our trainees. Trainees are watching us closely, both our verbal and nonverbal communications. They are not only asking, "How do I learn and apply your medical knowledge?" but also, "How do you look at the patient and others?" "Where do you sit?" "What are your expressions and word choices?" "What is your tone of voice?" "How do you give bad news?" "How do you handle emotions?" and "How do you talk about the patient when the patient is not present?" Trainees listen to our tone and read between the lines. They watch our body language. They are listening and watching when we don't think they are. It is clear that while we mentor them, they learn from us through observational learning.

Certainly, I have seen both good and bad communication skills in our superiors. In terms of bad communication, most of this has been speaking past a patient, or broaching a difficult topic without much tact or warning.

—Medical student

Do medical students come into the medical education system as better communicators than when they finish their training? Often, patients seem more satisfied after interacting with a first-year medical student than with a resident or even a mid-career physician. Furthermore, a medical student will gather more information from the patient while giving the patient more of a sense of caring than anyone else on the medical team. Students generally have more time with each patient than other team members, but often they also appear to have more curiosity and empathy as well as the ability to communicate those traits. We know that empathy and perhaps our communication skills wain during our training. This may be due in part to our physical and emotional exhaustion. But it may also be due to our lack of role models and specific discussions about displaying empathy and excellent communication between physicians and patients. And, unfortunately, after our medical training, we may never fully regain the ability to sit and to be present and curious about another person in a clinical setting as we did when we were first-year medical students. Once in practice, we may not have the time or the interest in assessing or improving our communication styles. Once we become "doctors" and they become "patients," we enter an arena rife with miscommunication and unsatisfying interactions. Perhaps the first-year medical students realize that the patient on the table could be their mother or sibling, or could even be them, and that is what helps them talk to the patients sincerely and with empathy.

Questions to Ask Yourself While Students and Residents Follow You

- Are you reading the patient's chart and becoming fully knowledgeable about the patient beforehand?
- Are you knocking on the patient's door first and waiting until the patient says "come in" before entering?
- Do you remain calm, focused, caring, and ready to listen to and learn from the patient?
- Do you shake hands, sit down, and make eye contact with the patient?
- Do you allow the patient to finish talking and not interrupt?
- Are you asking about the patient's fears and expectations?
- Do you check in with your patients to make sure they understand what you are saying?
- Do you answer their questions and then make sure they understand your answer?
- Do you allow the trainees to come with you during difficult encounters and when you need to break bad news?
- Are you displaying empathy?
- Are you actively listening? ("What I hear you saying is. . . .")
- While talking about the patient with staff or the trainee, are you respectful and nonjudgmental?
- How effectively do you work on the patient's behalf?
- Do you acknowledge and address the patient's emotions?
- Do you create a collaborative and caring environment for the patient?
- Are you always respectful of patients, family members, staff, and trainees?
- Are you successful in making sure the patient has no more questions?
- Are you summarizing and offering closure with each patient?

You may have witnessed the same scenario I have on teaching rounds at the hospital when the junior member of the team imitates the senior member. If medical students or interns perceive someone on their team (often the senior resident, chief resident, or attending) as being the most knowledgeable, then no matter how poorly the senior clinician communicates, the trainees begin to imitate that person's communication style. If the third-year resident speaks in a quiet low monotone manner (and much too quickly) while presenting information to the group, then the medical students will start to do the same. If the chief resident is abrupt, avoids shaking hands with the patient, and is only slightly engaged with patients, then others will follow suit. I have seen this time and time again. Whether it is with presentations or interactions with patients, everyone on the team starts to imitate the senior person— and not always the best communicator.

In teaching students and residents to ask specific questions, do we end up forcing them to ask leading questions as part of the history assessment? In trying to obtain certain clinical information, are we unknowingly encouraging the trainee to ask leading closed-ending questions instead of open-ended questions? Are we discouraging letting the patients tell their own story in their own words to the trainee? In asking physicians to see patients more quickly while they type into a computer, are we forcing them to become interrogators instead of caregivers practicing active listening and shared dialogue?

How can we better mentor our trainees about their communication styles and skills? To improve our trainees' communication skills, we must first acknowledge our "hidden curriculum"—how we are modeling behavior, communication, and interpersonal skills for our trainees. Second, we should assess and improve our own communication skills. And finally, we should create comprehensive, integrated, and ongoing communication programs for trainees and faculty together.

I have often thought about what the differences in patient satisfaction scores would be between the patient interviewed by a first-year medical student on their very first day of medical school, someone who is ten or fifteen years out of training, and a senior clinician who is thirty or forty years out of training. My guess is that the medical student might receive the highest scores for authenticity, empathy, listening, and overall attentive human dialogue. The senior clinician might score positive reviews as well, but I worry about all the years in between. What happens to our communication skills during training and practice? Medical school, residency, and the first few years of practice do not train us to communicate well with people. In fact, our training years may do just the opposite by putting a greater distance between us and our patients through shrinking our time and our relationship with patients, putting computer screens between us, and not having systems in place that support us, our patients, and patient–physician relationships, dialogue, and collaboration.

Furthermore, studies have shown that it is not easy to measure how our trainees are retaining communication skills. While we might congratulate ourselves on communication sessions we teach in medical school or residency, there are still no studies showing a relationship between the scores students or even residents may achieve on various communications skills assessments and their skills or their patients' satisfaction scores once they are in practice.

Advice for Teaching Communication Skills to Trainees

1. Listen and observe them: they will show and tell you what they need.
2. Realize they are learning more from observing what you do than from what you say.

3. Realize that by the time you are working with them, medical training may have worsened their inherently great communications skills.

4. Watch their verbal and nonverbal communication skills.

5. Observe their emotional cues with you and with patients.

6. Remind them to think of themselves or their family members on the table someday.

7. Encourage them to discuss their own thoughts and feelings about communicating with patients and peers.

8. Encourage them to continue their communications training throughout their careers.

Further Reading

Adrienne Boissy and Timothy Gilligan, *Communication the Cleveland Clinic Way: How to Drive a Relationship-Centered Strategy for Superior Patient Experience* (New York: McGraw-Hill, 2016).

Roman W. DeSanctis, *On Being a Physician* (Middletown, DE: @Roman W. DeSanctis, 2018).

Jennifer Fong Ha et al., "Doctor-Patient Communication: A Review," *Ochsner Journal*, 2010;10:38–43.

Wendy Leebov and Carla Rotering, *The Language of Caring Guide for Physicians: Communication Essentials for Patient-Centered Care*, 2nd edition (Language of Caring, LLC, 2014).

David Matsumoto, Mark G. Frank, and Hyi Sung Hwang, *Nonverbal Communication: Science and Application* (Thousand Oaks, CA: Sage Publications, 2013).

Joe Navarro, *What Every Body Is Saying: An Ex-FBI Agent's Guide to Speed Reading People* (New York: Harper Collins, 2014).

References

1. Roman W. DeSanctis, *On Being a Physician* (Middletown, DE: @Roman W. DeSanctis, 2018).

2. A. Boissy, A. K. Windover, D. Bokar et al., "Communication Skills Training for Physicians Improves Patient Satisfaction," *Journal of General Internal Medicine*, 2016;31(7):755–761.

3. The Joint Commission. Retrieved from: https://jointcommission.org https://www.jointcommission.org/assets/1/23/jconline_April_29_15.pdf.

4. The Joint Commission, "Facts about Patient-Centered Communication," January 6, 2019. Retrieved from https://www.jointcommission.org/facts_about_patient-centered_communications/.

5. The Joint Commission, "Health Equity Portal." Retrieved from https://www.jointcommission.org/topics/health_equity.aspx.

6. L. Kettleson, K. Cook, and B. Kennedy, *The HCAHPS Handbook 2: Tactics to Improve Quality and the Patient Experience*, 2nd edition (Pensacola, FL: Fire Starter Publishing, 2014).

7. A. Boissy and T. Gilligan, *Communication the Cleveland Clinic Way: How to Drive a Relationship-Centered Strategy for Superior Patient Experience* (New York: McGraw-Hill, 2016).

8. Agency for Healthcare Research and Quality. Retrieved from https://www.ahrq.gov.

9. H. B. Beckman and R. M. Frankel, "The Effect of Physician Behavior on the Collection of Data," *Annals of Internal Medicine*, 1984;101:692–696.

10. M. Marvel, R. Epstein, K. Flowers, and H. Beckman, "Soliciting the Patient's Agenda: Have We Improved?" *JAMA: The Journal of the American Medical Association*, 1999;281(3):283–287.

11. W. Langewitz, M. Denz, M. A. Keller, A. Kiss, S. Ruttimann, and B. Wossmer, "Spontaneous Talking Time at Start of Consultation in Outpatient Clinic: Cohort Study," *BMJ*, 2002;325(7366):682–683.

12. "Harris Poll Survey Finds Patients Want a Deeper Digital Connection with Their Doctor," *Business Wire*, April 6, 2015. Retrieved from: https://www.businesswire.com/news/home/20150406005190/en/Harris-Poll-Survey-Finds-Patients-Deeper-Digital.

13. D. Toft, February 10, 2018. Retrieved from: https://dougtoft.net/2018/02/10/the-intimacy-of-shared-silence/.

14. Aristotle and W. R. Roberts, *Rhetoric* (Dover Thrift Editions, 2012).

15. R. C. Lorenzetti, C. H. Mitch Jacques, and C. Donovan et al. "Managing Difficult Encounters: Understanding Physician, Patient, and Situational Factors," *American Family Physician*, 2013;87(6):419–425.

16. ACLS Certification Institute. Retrieved from https://acls.com/free-resources/knowledge-base/bls-articles/resuscitation-team-dynamics.

17. A. Fitzgerald Chase, "Team Communication in Emergencies: Simple Strategies for Staff." Retrieved from http://www.zoll.com/codecommunicationsnewsletter/ccnl04_10/ZollTeamCommunications04_10.pdf.

18. J. K. Burgoon, L. K. Guerrero, and K. Floyd, *Nonverbal Communication* (Boston: Allyn and Bacon, 2009).

19. P. Philippot, R. Feldman, and E. Coats, "The Role of Nonverbal Behavior in Clinical Settings," in P. Philippot, R. Feldman, and E. Coats E, editors, *Nonverbal Behavior in Clinical Settings* (New York: Oxford University Press, 2003), pp. 3–13.

2

Digital Communication

Introduction

How do we keep the human presence and perspective, as well as humanity, inside the personal conversations that take place in medicine? As physicians, our ability to listen, empathize, and communicate our observations, reasoning, and knowledge in a thoughtful way is our most vital tool. While the electronic universe has given us unbelievable advantages, it does have its downsides. Even those working within the profession of medicine may sometimes appear to be more worried about efficiency, data analytics, and the use of the latest technology than the comfort and care of humans. Perhaps we know we should be talking more and typing less, and observing longer, listening deeper, and reducing the time we spend clicking, tweeting, and blogging. We need to remember to utilize other opportunities to gather knowledge and connect with each other than through an electronic screen. But how can we compete with the virtual, seductive, endless, immediate, and often essential information now available at our fingertips? Once we have the knowledge and expertise we need, what will prompt us to close our computer screens, turn away from our electronic devices, and open our eyes, ears, and hearts as humans and as caring doctors? Or can we devise ways to retain our compassion and care as we hold the computer in one hand and the patient in the other?

There are few aspects of society, including clinical medicine, still untouched by digital communication and the Internet. It seems harder and harder to think of daily interactions or common transactions we all have, inside or outside the clinic, that are not conducted, facilitated, augmented, or wholly reliant on computer screens. Try to identify pockets of your life untouched by the Internet, and you might find a challenge. There are very few service economies we use, or personal and professional interactions we have, including those in healthcare, that are free from the Internet and independent of electronic screens.

It would seem that the important and intimate conversations in a doctor's office or at the bedside should be one of the last refuges to provide private face-to-face discourse between two humans, free of the distraction and the distance of the computer. But, as we all know, that is changing. From computers in the exam room to electronic medical records, to email exchanges and texting with patients, computers are ever present in the delivery of healthcare. Imagine removing all of the familiar aspects of human communication, from verbal to nonverbal cues, facial expressions, body language, attentive listening, clear articulation, important pauses, observations, empathy, natural vocal tones, eye contact, human touch, and the use of instinctive physical gestures. When you remove the human elements of traditional communication, you will unfortunately find yourself in a world where more and more people, including physicians and patients, interact, gather information, and express themselves daily through technology. Welcome to the world of digital communications.

Of course, information technology has revolutionized medicine, and the advantages for patients and physicians are numerous. Through patient computer portals, patients can now look at their lab results and treatments and ask relevant questions; physicians can respond quickly to emailed questions; and patients can inform themselves about surgery by watching online videos, see their x-rays, and have more informative conversations with their doctors. Apps can monitor our physiology; robots can deliver medication and perform surgery; and artificial intelligence is playing a bigger role in the analysis of complex healthcare data.

Today, patients show physicians pictures on their cell phones of the rash they had last week or an x-ray from another hospital. A retired college professor related a story to me about how his cell phone changed his spouse's scheduled lumbar puncture (spinal tap) in an emergency department. He recalled, "The docs were not aware that she had had major spinal surgery in the past with a metal plate in the region of L4-L5." But her record and x-ray were on his cell phone. Once he showed the doctors the x-ray of his wife's spine (Figure 2.1), it altered their approach. She immediately went down for a fluoroscopically guided lumbar puncture instead of the doctors performing it at the bedside. Fortunately, all went well, and the results from the lumbar puncture were negative.

The quick adoption and global reach of this relatively embryonic technology of Internet communications are astounding—from cell phone data exchanges to live streaming interactive videos and other electronic forms of communication. The impact and influence on individuals, societies, and professions, including medicine, may exceed some of the most significant media inventions over the last 600 years, such as Johannes Gutenberg's printing press of the

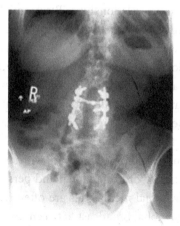

Figure 2.1 X-ray showing spinal fusion hardware.

15th century, Samuel Morse's telegraph and Alexander Graham Bell's telephone of the 19th century, and commercial television of the 20th century.

Today, whether our chosen form of social communication is a blog, a tweet, a text, or an email, our electronic correspondence tends to be brief, unedited, unfiltered, and public. The speed with which we send and expect to receive electronic signals and manage electronic data is no less than astounding. We don't seem to mind that our digital communication is more of a brief monologue and less a thoughtful human dialogue. For some, "likes" and "dislikes" or illustrations of thumbs up or down seem to have replaced any in-depth response or true discourse. Tweets have become the equivalent of a sandwich board or political placard. Blogs are how we stand and shout in the public square. Instagram is how we share a picture of what we are eating, seeing, or wearing. There seems to be little time or space for deep reflection or thought. Respectful deliberations are not expected or encouraged. The number of followers one has on Twitter or elsewhere has become the measure of success for some.

For many in a professional sphere, including doctors, email, texting, and instant messaging define workloads and often professional and personal relationships. Electronic medical records (EMRs), where we click boxes of current problems and diagnostic codes instead of writing lengthy and unique details of important clinical observations and findings, have become one of the most time-consuming and cumbersome aspects of physician communications. Conversations with our patients, students, residents, and colleagues have been replaced with typing on electronic keyboards and into our smart phones.

Many physicians have jumped on board with social media, where they can have a variety of professional and personal interactions. But unfortunately, social media sites are often where the conversation is more of a global broadcast between disparate individuals at distant computers using keystrokes, cameras, graphics, microphones, and other multimedia tools. Emails and texts have joined blogs, posts, and tweets as the preferred transmission between individuals, organizations, and institutions. Some are peddling their opinions, positions, wares, and services. Some messages are disguised as important communiques, while information and personal data are gathered, stored, analyzed, and commodified by governments, institutions, or corporations.

As users of digital communications even in the medical sphere, we seem to have lowered our expectations for privacy, security, confidentiality, quality, accuracy and accountability. Somehow even as doctors, we seem to ignore the impact of technology on our minds, attentions spans, opinions, gullibility, reasoning, decision-making, knowledge levels, and communication skills. The comfort and familiarity of face-to-face conversations, as well as other human connections and interactions, may be at risk, never mind our ability to focus on one task or an in-depth endeavor at a time.

We have adapted to the electronic universe even in medicine. Our behavior, our personal interactions, and our expectations for access and processing of information, as well as our communication style, have all been altered at least while we are using digital communications (which now seems like most of the time). Many physicians and patients may even feel more comfortable, confident, and in control when communicating through screens than in person.

There is no doubt that digital communication comes with remarkable speed and the ability to travel across unlimited geographic boundaries, providing access to staggering amounts of data and new ways to locate, analyze, and display those data as never before.

Digital communication in medicine is certainly here to stay, assuming a bigger role in our daily clinical lives and our patients' lives; patients are reminded to take their medicine by electronic messaging, and they are recording their electrocardiograms with their smart phones and sending us electronic diaries of their moods, blood sugar levels, heart rates, and blood pressures. Patients are Skyping with their doctors. Doctors are using various forms of technology to assess trends in physiologic markers and to predict clinical outcomes.

This chapter will take a closer look at the different methods that physicians, patients, and other medical professionals are using to communicate and interact in social and professional digital electronic spheres.

Social Media

Today, more than three billion people, almost half of the world's population, use the Internet. According to Statista, an online statistics market research and business intelligence portal, 77% of Americans have a social media profile, and 2.34 billion people worldwide use social media.[1] The reality and perceptions of social media content are unique, unparalleled, and often unaligned. Whether you use Facebook, Twitter, LinkedIn, Reddit, Snapchat, Instagram, blogs, organizational websites, or other online social media sites, you quickly learn that the content is fleeting yet permanent; virtual yet real; private yet public; anonymous yet discoverable—all unusual combinations in the history of communications. This is true particularly regarding physician-to-patient, physician-to-physician, and physician-to-public communications. The number of users of social media is globally pervasive. As of 2018, some of the most popular electronic social media websites in the blogosphere were Facebook (2.23 billion users), YouTube (1.9 billion), WhatsApp (1.5 billion), Facebook Messenger (1.3 billion), WeChat (1.06 billion), Instagram (1.0 billion), Tumblr (23 million), Twitter (67million), Snapchat (186 million), and Pinterest (250 million). LinkedIn reported 500 million users in 2018.[2]

Social media platforms are the public square where anyone, anywhere with access to the Internet can participate. In this sphere, vast amounts of medical information also exists in the form of health news, clinical instructional videos, physician blogs and tweets, continuing medical education (CME) podcasts, patient support groups, and physician rating sites. Online information from almost every major medical publication, organization, and academic institution is updated daily, hourly, or even by the minute.

Patients often turn to social media for medical information and advice or to find a doctor or a patient support group, and physicians, hospitals, and healthcare organizations have taken note. Half of physician practices (53%) now have a Facebook page.[3] Most of the major hospitals have a presence on Facebook and Twitter or other social media sites (Figure 2.2). Of the 5624 hospitals in the United States, 26% participate in social media.[4] Of the approximately 1500 hospitals nationwide that have an online presence, Facebook is the most popular social media website—just as it is in the general public.[5] After the Mayo Clinic started using social media, its podcast listeners rose by 76,000 according to the Infographics Archive.[6]

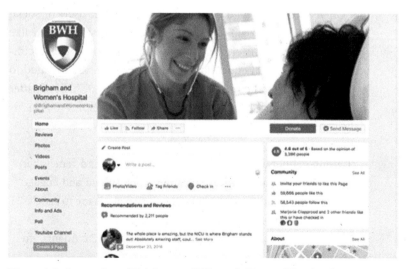

Figure 2.2 Screenshot of Brigham and Women's Hospital Facebook page.

The top ten hospitals on social media include the Mayo Clinic, Cleveland's MetroHealth System, Baylor Health Care System, Rush University Medical Center, Oregon Health and Science University, Vanderbilt Health, and The Mount Sinai Hospital.[7]

Today, most hospitals, academic institutions, and professional organizations have special departments and assigned professionals who direct how they use and engage in social media; institutional leaders perceive the benefits for their overall missions and of staying connected to the public. Individual physicians who participate in social media perceive the benefits as "forwarding their career or research endeavors, self-improvement through reading others' tweets and keeping up with the literature, increasing their reach, (i.e., their audience), and providing a space for them to openly express their opinions," according to one study by Campbell et al.[8] Just as it has in other areas of our society, social media has allowed patients, providers, and institutions to break down traditional barriers to communication and increase the options for, access to, and speed of connections we can make with each other.

Dr. Adam Cifu, Professor of Medicine and general internist at the University of Chicago, is one of the two billion users of social media around the world (Figure 2.3). But he may not seem like your typical Twitter user. Dr. Cifu divides his time between clinical practice, medical education, and scholarly research related to evidence-based medicine. He also has more than 7,788 Twitter followers as of April 2019. For him, Twitter is a helpful tool in his daily professional life.

> Tweeting about articles helps me to synthesize and remember them. Tweeting about ideas helps me process them and engage with others for online brainstorming. It also alerts me to articles I would have missed.
>
> —Dr. Adam Cifu

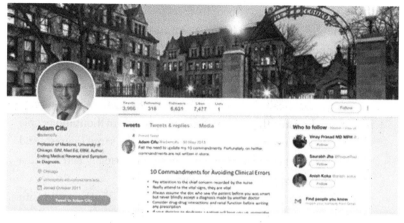

Figure 2.3 Screenshot of Dr. Adam Cifu's Twitter page.

Dr. Cifu is also the author of a textbook and a book for the lay public: *Symptoms to Diagnosis: An Evidence-Based Guide* and *Ending Medical Reversal: Improving Outcomes Saving Lives*. He tried to use Twitter twice since 2011, but finally "got it right" in 2015 when he decided to limit his audience to those who were interested in clinical and academic medicine. Like other professionals, he does not necessarily want to hear what someone had for dinner or where they went on vacation; he only wants to discuss issues related to internal medicine. Twitter has introduced Dr. Cifu to "thousands of valuable, virtual colleagues." Since 2015, he has written thousands of posts. He cannot see giving up his global Twitter audience of professional colleagues, where he averages one hundred posts a month. "Right now, I have incorporated it into my professional life to enough of a degree that giving it up would honestly feel like giving up colleagues," he says.

Dr. Cifu does not see any downsides to using social media, other than it takes time. He says he leaves his Twitter account open on his desk all day while he is working and seeing patients or going to meetings. It does not interfere with his work and gives him an ongoing connection to like-minded colleagues.

It is a weird society of people who I feel attached to in some way though I am absolutely not attached to because most of them are anonymous. . . . I have no idea who they really are. . . . I am a general internist, my section of internists are about 40 people who are very close colleagues I work with clinically and collaborate academically but that is 40 people of whom 5 are passionate about the same things I am. Here are a couple of thousand people [Twitter followers] who because we have the same interests and talk about the same things on Twitter that usually extends to a much larger group. It is very helpful.

—Dr. Adam Cifu

As the definition and reach of social media continue to evolve, so do the use and potential misuse by organizations and individuals in the profession. With the sheer amount of daily new medical information; the need for accurate point-of-care updates; the public's appetite for health news; organizations' pursuit of marketing, branding, fundraising, and self-promotion; and the allure of data analytics, all combined with the speed, function, and expanse of the World Wide Web, we have created either a perfect universe of information or a perfect storm of misinformation—or perhaps both, depending on your point of view.

The term "social media" first appeared in 2004. Since that time, and with the growing electronic universe, the definition continues to evolve. The *Oxford English Living Dictionary* defines social media as the "websites and applications that enable users to create and share content or to participate in social networking." The *Merriam-Webster Dictionary* defines social media as "forms of electronic communication, such as websites for social networking and microblogging, through which users create online communities to share information, ideas, personal messages, and other content such as videos." Wikipedia uses more than 17,000 words and a bibliography of more than 200 references to define social media.

Physicians use social media for professional networking, clinical education, research collaboration, organizational skills training, patient care, patient engagement and interaction, publicity, and public health promotion, according to medical writer Lee Ventola.[9] According to Ventola, more than 90% of physicians use some form of social media for personal activities, whereas only 65% use these sites for professional reasons. Nearly one-third of physicians have reported participating in social networks; and both personal and professional use of social media by physicians is increasing.[9]

Physicians' use of the Internet and social media appears to parallel the rest of the population in numbers, with the majority of adults using some form of social media, including Facebook, Twitter, or other applications.

Social media use falls into three broad categories: creation, curation, and consumption, according to, co-founder and Managing Partner of Asentech. Bhaskar believes that very few social media users are actually creating original content, while most are either occasionally commenting on others' posts or passively viewing what is "published" on the site.[10] Bhaskar writes, "Approximately 1% of healthcare professionals using social media are content producers, creating and publishing original content. These physicians are creating blogs, forums, and information-sharing websites that provide information to e-Patients and other healthcare professionals. Another 9% engage with others on social media by commenting on posts and participating in group discussions or online chats. Content curation activities include identifying and sharing useful information or links with followers or other members of an online community. Finally, 90% of physicians are social media consumers. These individuals use the Internet and social media to find and read relevant information related to their patients and practice."

Social Media and Mainstream Medical Media

It is not just access and availability that physicians and patients are interested in, but also accuracy and accountability. They both want evidence-based information, quality research findings, and clinical guidelines from reputable resources.

Physicians use online resources to access medical news and updates, clinical and diagnostic tools, drug databases, and patient information, according to Bhaskar. Physicians have also become accustomed to reading professional and academic journals online, doing CME activities electronically, and accessing clinical points of care from a computer screen on their desktop computer, tablet, or even cell phone. Social media has become the superhighway where some of this data are publicized, reposted, debated, and discussed.

For nearly a decade, most traditional media organizations, including medical publishing organizations and medical institutions, have climbed aboard the social media bandwagon. Most organizations have Facebook and Twitter accounts, including the *New York Times*, the Cleveland Clinic, and the National Institutes of Health. Even the venerable two-hundred-year-old *New England Journal of Medicine (NEJM)* has a Facebook page (Figure 2.4). In 2017, the *NEJM* reached one million followers on Facebook, more than the number of their individual paid subscribers.

"It is important for us to be where our audience is, and social media allows us to do this," said Jennifer Zeis, Manager of Communications and Media Relations at the *NEJM* in 2018. Zeis knows that social media works because when the *NEJM* posts an article or image on social media, it drives readers to the *NEJM* main website where the original articles and other peer-reviewed primary content have been published. As with other activity on the Internet, social media users can be tracked with "clicks" and "likes," comments, and other data (Figure 2.5).

The *NEJM* Executive Editor and Online Editor, Edward W. Campion, who has worked at the *NEJM* for nearly three decades,

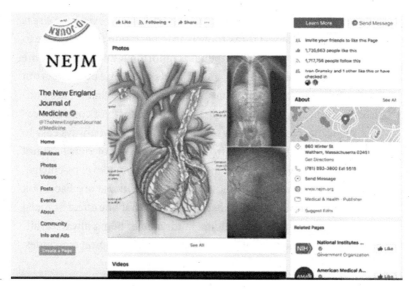

Figure 2.4 Screenshot of the *New England Journal of Medicine* Facebook page.

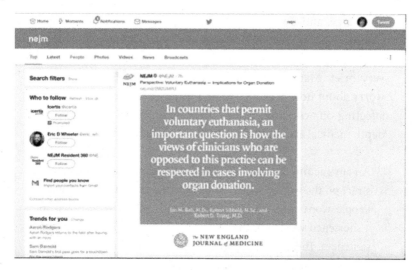

In countries that permit voluntary euthanasia, an important question is how the views of clinicians who are opposed to this practice can be respected in cases involving organ donation.

Figure 2.5 Screenshot of the *New England Journal of Medicine* Twitter page.

believes that using social media is necessary because everyone else is there. Campion says, "I think there is an expectation that you have to have a presence there. If not, then it is ignoring it and there is some opportunity there." Campion adds, "It gets our name out, it gets out some of the news content, what we are doing and what we are publishing." But Campion says while this modern form of communication seems necessary in today's digital world, it is not always easy to know why. "What it achieves from a business point of view I am not sure other than visibility and awareness and some level of engagement," adds Campion, "you know off the site, those are Facebook users, they are not our subscribers. . . . I think that one effect of social media plays into the whole digital landscape of being always available, 24/7, free and kind of fast and superficial," Campion concludes.

An Expanding or Contracting Universe?

Social media options for individuals and organizations continue to enlarge, and Twitter has increased its space to 280 characters. (A character on Twitter is defined as a letter, number, punctuation mark, or space.) But most online communication still tends to be very brief. Many individuals, including *NEJM* Editor Campion, worry about how brief electronic messages, in every form, may be affecting our comprehension, consumption, and retention of in-depth medical articles and scientific information.

> An abstract used to be thought of as the short form. But an abstract on the web or social media or email or twitter is too long. People won't read something that long. It has come down to a shortened version of the title and the web blurb which is two sentences. The attention span is shorter and of course the screens are getting smaller. Most people, especially younger generations are reading on the small screens, on their phones. Ten years ago, that was kind of unthinkable.
>
> —Edward W. Campion

The main benefit of having a social media presence for institutions like the *NEJM* may be dissemination, marketing, and discussion of their articles in the electronic public sphere. But there are also other advantages when it comes to their global reach to readers. "For us, the main benefit [of social media] is just awareness. A lot of people see what is in the journal. It doesn't lead to deep engagement. But a broad awareness including an international audience," according to Campion, "The Journal's audience is hugely international, and internet and digital delivery and Twitter and Facebook and our million plus people on the email list, allow for more an instant connection with no delay. In the old days, we would send out paper copies that never got there at least in remote places." Unfortunately, what is often of most interest on social media, is not the lead article or an important ground-breaking clinical finding in the *Journal*.

> It is true that the things that have gone viral on social media have been pretty trivial, Oscar the cat who could sense when someone was dying, the media and social media got onto that. A parasite crawling out of someone's ear or across an eyeball or something like that are the ones that get a huge amount of attention. It has kind of made for some voyeurism. Social media is part voyeurism.
>
> —Edward W. Campion

So, if social media is largely voyeuristic and it may or may not be prompting individuals to read longer articles or engage in in-depth conversations, what are the tangible benefits and the real purpose? Besides a way to republish articles and drive traffic to an institution's website, what other purpose does social media serve? Is it really education, collaboration, and discussion, or a place to grab quick bits of data as we need them? Is it often more advertising, marketing, and promotion disguised as information or articles? Is it a way for Facebook or other institutions and individuals to collect, exploit, and monetize our data? For individual physicians, is there any role or specific advantage to using social media—or is it a vast waste of time and distraction with little benefit? What exactly is the signal-to-noise ratio of social media for doctors? Only each individual physician can answer those questions for himself or herself.

The Twitter World of Medicine

If you search for doctors you know or know of, you may be surprised how many are using Twitter. It seems that one of the ultimate goals of having a Twitter account is how many followers you accumulate. As one editorial cartoon by Randy Glasbergen points out in the dialogue between two men: "It is difficult to place a value on my company. Which is worth more, a million shareholders or a million Twitter followers?" The same might be said by physicians with Twitter accounts.

After following and reading various Twitter accounts, you may wonder if there is an inverse relationship between the number of a person's Twitter followers and the uniqueness, usefulness, and strength of their content, depending on what you are looking for. A wide range of physicians, besides University of Chicago internist Adam Cifu, have Twitter accounts. Here are just a few physicians and the number of Twitter followers each had as of April 2019:

- **Dr. Eric Topol**, former chairman of cardiovascular medicine at the Cleveland Clinic, now founder and director of the Scripps Translational Science Institute, and awarded a $207 million grant for precision medicine initiative in 2016 (158,000 Twitter followers)
- **Dr. Siddhartha Mukherjee**, oncologist, writer, and winner of the 2011 Pulitzer Prize for *The Emperor of All Maladies: A Biography of Cancer* (39,400 Twitter followers)
- **Dr. Francis Collins**, the director of the National Institutes of Medicine (103,000 Twitter followers)

- Dr. Jennifer Ashton, obstetrician-gynecologist and ABC News Chief Medical Correspondent (72,300 Twitter followers)
- Dr. Kevin Pho, primary care doctor in New Hampshire, physician, and author (157,000 Twitter followers)
- Dr. Travis Stork, emergency room doctor and host of television show, *The Doctors* (169,000 Twitter followers)

In 2017, Twitter expanded its word limit from 140 to 280 characters, but according to Jack Dorsey, CEO of Twitter, the length of the average tweet has not gone up since the character limit change was implemented. The average tweet is about 50 characters—and the average number of words is just 15, not exactly an extensive missive. The most popular activity for physicians on Twitter seems to be tweeting while reposting an article. Unlike traditional media outlets with large staffs who publish numerous articles and original content regularly, many social media users (including physician bloggers and Tweeters) have found that producing original content is challenging, laborious, and time-consuming, and as some in daily journalism would say, next to impossible to continue to "feed the daily news beast." It is often much easier just to repost someone else's article and make a quick comment than to write and post your own original material.

Many Twitter doctors engage in a wide range of activities from commenting on an article, cartoon, or image to reposting their own published articles or updates from their institutions. Some physicians post broadcast links to medical conferences or videos or try to engage their audience with a question or political statement. On one day in 2018, Dr. Ashton from ABC News was looking for people who had recently been diagnosed with bronchitis, presumably for her ABC News show. On other days she reposted videos from the *Good Morning America* television show explaining the new FDA guidelines on e-cigarettes, a new flu strain, and information about superbugs. On another day in 2018, acclaimed author, clinician and researcher Dr. Jerome

Groopman reposted an op-ed article by Tom Brokaw written in the *New York Times*. Dr. Groopman echoed Brokaw's sentiment and posted his own message, "at a time of rising xenophobia, people with anti-immigrant prejudice should consider that immigrants and their offspring might save their lives." In September of 2018, Dr. Eric Topol retweeted a *NEJM* article concerning the association of low-dose aspirin and all cause mortality and then Dr. Groopman retweeted Dr. Topol's comments as well as his own. Groopman wrote, "Another important finding that argues against coercive quality metrics—every study limitations, and risk/benefit analysis has a subjective core. Better to debate data, honor patient preference and await superior research than top down mandates." It was a brief medical discussion between two academic clinicians in less than 280 characters. For many physicians, social media has become the way to converse about important ideas, articles, and observations. For others, it is a way to begin an important conversation or "get something off their chest," or for a way to market themselves or their book, work, research article, or institution.

Dr. Aditi Nerurkar, an integrative medicine specialist, Instructor in Medicine at Harvard Medical School, primary care doctor at Beth Israel Hospital in Boston, and writer, describes her social media use as "a 'living business card' for media to find me." For Dr. Nerurkar and others, social media allows them to update and post their writings, observations, research, and press coverage; Twitter, Facebook, Instagram, Indeed and other online social media venues offer these and other opportunities for physcians who are interested.

Physician-to-Patient Digital Communication

Physicians and healthcare institutions are quickly realizing that social media can be an efficacious way to educate, communicate with, and attract patients. Patients use social media to find medical information and advice, hospitals and providers, and even other patients. There are myriad ways institutions are captivating and educating patients through social media.

Dr. Joseph Dearani, Chair of the Department of Cardiovascular Surgery at the Mayo Clinic, specializes in the repair of pediatric and adult congenital heart surgery, including Ebstein's anomaly. He has created a Facebook page for patients so that they not only can watch a video about cardiac problems and therapeutic procedures but also can hear about, and meet, other families who have been through similar problems and interventions. Facebook helps him and his department inform patients and families before he meets them in person. According to Lee Aase, director of the Mayo Clinic Social Media Network, the electronic consumer space of Facebook and other social media sites "are not replacements for a visit with the doctor," but, if used properly, can be "effective tools to educate and engage patients." By the time that patients and their families meet with the doctor, they may feel like they know the doctor from watching a video presentation. They may understand more about their diagnosis from watching the diagrams, explanations, and patients discussing their treatment on the website. The online information may prompt patients and their families to formulate their questions and concerns before their first visit; and it may make the exchange of information in the face-to-face meeting easier and more productive.

The Mayo Clinic has also used Facebook and other social media sites in various ways to promote public health programs and increase awareness about important health issues such as colonoscopy and other health screenings. The Mayo Clinic has produced programs such as a "live stream" colonoscopy to promote screening colonoscopies. The Mayo Clinic's transplantation center posts blogs to educate the public about living organ donation and helps connect potential living donors and recipients (Figure 2.6).

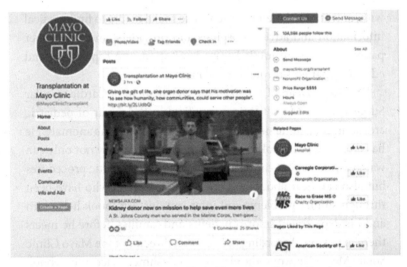

Figure 2.6 Screenshot of the Mayo Clinic Transplant Center Facebook page.

Social media platforms and other online medical information can help patients understand their condition and be more involved with their treatment; overall, it encourages patients to play a more active role in their healthcare. But according to Ivan De Martino in an article published in the *Current Review of Musculoskeletal Medicine* in 2017, "In this way, patients are not passive consumers of health information." But he warns that the electronic medium is not without risks: "it is difficult to control or regulate the sources and their quality, and bad or misleading information can be detrimental for patients as well as influence their confidence on physicians and their mutual relationship."[11]

Clearly, the institutions, professional organizations, and individuals engaging with social media directly determine the quality of the content they post. The problem comes when patients are searching for important or even life-saving information and don't know how to find reputable sources or recognize established and credible organizations. Just like with all information online, there are broad-ranging concerns about quality, authenticity, and accountability of medical information online. In 2018, Facebook deleted 583 million fake accounts, more than 25% of the 2.2 million monthly active users. How can patients or anyone be certain that what they are seeing or reading online is true or is actually from the person or institution supposedly behind the post?

Risks of Social Media

User-generated content by physicians or any other social media users, such as text posts, comments, articles, photos, videos, and online interactions, are the "lifeblood of social media"; however, any information on any social media platform is not without risks. "There are concerns about the security, privacy, and confidentiality of the personal health-related information shared on these social platforms; the quality and accuracy of the information shared; and the credibility of the individuals who post medical advices and tips," writes Ivan De Martino. Professional organizations and other institutions have begun to develop guidelines for healthcare professionals regarding social media. (There is a list of guidelines at the end of this chapter and a list of resources concerning social media and digital communications.)

While social media sites can promote individual and public health, as well as professional development and advancement, according to Ventola, "when used negligently, the privacy and security risks concerning health care information are very real." That is why, if you engage in social media, it is critical to stay up to date on the guidelines provided by medical-legal professionals, healthcare organizations, medical societies, and others to help you avoid problems.

Social Media and Medical Conferences

Each year, there seem to be new communication uses for social media. There is an increased growth and rapid use of Twitter, Facebook, and other platforms by healthcare providers attending medical conferences who want to communicate with their colleagues, patients, and the public. According to hematologist-oncologist Dr. Naveen Pemmaraju of MD Anderson Cancer Center, there is a growing amount of research in this area demonstrating an increasing interest among physicians on how to use social media for consumption of educational material and how to generate and contribute original content based on one's interests and expertise. It is not uncommon for physicians sitting at medical conferences to update their Twitter posts from their laptops and Facebook pages from their cell phones.

Dr. Pemmaraju writes, "Hematologists/oncologists are engaging regularly in one of the most common forms of social media, Twitter, during major medical conferences, for purposes of debate, discussion, and real-time evaluation of the data being presented."[12]

Providing the ability to communicate real-time updates and information from conferences helps physicians inform and engage colleagues and the public. It also may serve as a "note-taking service" for the physicians themselves while they are busy posting and commenting on the information presented at the meeting in real time. They may field questions, initiate discussions, and post comments from their colleagues who are not physically in attendance at the medical conference.

In this way, the information presented at medical conferences is disseminated and publicized to a much broader audience at no added expense by the conference organizers. Yet there may be a loss of registration fees or control for conference administrators, since many who did not pay to attend the conference may be gaining immediate access to some of the information presented. For some conference organizers, it may be a win-lose situation: they are gaining publicity but losing attendance rates and some sense of command over their content distribution. But many medical conferences now charge for "electronic attendance" or access to full online video recordings after the conference and run their own blogs and posted discussions. Conferences are also upping their technology games by using live interactive polling and other electronic devices to keep their audiences engaged.

Physician Reviews and Ratings
on Social Media

The online physician ratings posted by patients are often one-way directed online messaging from anonymous individuals and hosted by organizational platforms. Much has been written about the pros and cons of online physician reviews. Many physicians are all too familiar with the sting of a negative online comment from an anonymous patient. Some sites allow for physicians to contest or respond to negative reviews and sometimes have them removed. Organizations can also offer advice on ways to respond to patient reviews, encourage patients to leave positive reviews, and help you improve your ratings. Many private companies and consultants now promise physicians and organizations help in managing their online reputations.

Regardless of the accuracy and authenticity of online physician reviews and ratings, patients still respond to them. One study by Carbonell published in 2018 in *Health Communication* found that patients' decisions about selecting a provider were influenced by online ratings—and the higher the number of users the more influence the social media cue had on patients' behavior in selecting and seeing a particular physician.[13]

> We found that the participants' likelihood to visit a physician varied with respect to the displayed physician characteristics on the platform. Importantly, after the recommendation of others was presented, participants' likelihood to visit the physician changed significantly. The participants' adjusted response was significantly closer to the recommendation coming from a higher number of users, which indicate that this online, social media cue influences our decision to visit physicians.
>
> —Guillemo Carbonell

Often, physicians will be more likely to receive positive online ratings for individual skills such as competence, likeability, and character. Negative ratings are more likely to be related to their office staff interactions, billing, and office environment, according to an observational study by Chester J. Donnally III in 2018.[14] Apparently, a social media presence on Facebook, Twitter, and Instagram increases the number of ratings and comments, but not overall scores on physician review websites. "Understanding the factors that optimize a patient's overall experience with a physician is an important and emerging outcome measure for the future of patient-centered health care," according to Donnally.

Physicians and Patients: Uses of Social Media

1. Communication
   a. Physician to physician
   b. Physician to patient; patient to patient (virtual health communities; MDTALKS.com)
   c. Physician to the public
2. Education
   a. Physician to physician/resident/student
   b. Physician to patient/the public
3. Collaboration
   a. Physician to physician (clinical information)
   b. Physician researcher to researcher
   c. Clinical researcher to patient
4. Marketing
   a. Physician self-promotion
   b. Organizational promotion
   c. Issue promotion/disease awareness
   d. Public health information dissemination
   e. Fundraising

Physician Social Networking Websites

The social networks Sermo www.sermo.com and Doximity www.doximity.com are examples of physician-only social networking communities. They allow physicians to discuss topics ranging from reimbursement and board recertification to patient care and personal issues. Other online social networks for doctors include DailyRounds www.dailyrounds.org; QuantiaMD www.quantiamd.com; Among Doctors www.amoungdoctors.com; Figure1 www.Figure1.com; Incision Academy www.incision.care; Student Doctors Network www.studentdoctor.net; MomMD www.mommd.com; and Doctor's Choice www.doctorschoiceusa.com. The website communities promise to offer professional connections, crowdsourcing, career and personal advice, and other educational and professional resources. Some allow for use of pseudonyms for anonymity. Many promise protection of information and offer text and images that are compliant with the Health Insurance Portability and Accountability Act (HIPAA). Physicians are also using "private" or organizational social media sites for point-of-care information as well as for discussions of various clinical conundrums, research topics, and professional collaborations.

I signed up for a physician-only social network and shortly began receiving regular email invitations to take surveys for which I would be paid $25 to $80. To participate in any of the surveys, you first have to answer a number of questions about yourself and your practice before they determine whether you qualify to take the survey questions. As many of us now know, our data are now a major commodity. Perhaps there are various ways, besides traditional electronic advertising, that some of these websites are funding their enterprises.

Electronic support groups are popular for physicians, just as they are for patients. Physician Moms Group https://mypmg.com was founded in November 2014 by Dr. Hala Sabry. Today, more than 71,000 physicians of all specialties share, collaborate, and support each other in this open forum. Various topics are shared and discussed, including financial, medical, career, family, child-raising, and relationship advice. A colleague of mine from medical school uses Physician Moms Group daily through Facebook and says that reading the stories of other women physicians' lives and their stresses is supportive, collaborative, and "a fantastic way to support other women physicians who are moms."

As more physicians participate in various social media opportunities, and even the *NEJM* has a Facebook page and a Twitter account, the Mayo Clinic has developed a social media department of education and physician networking. The Mayo Clinic Social Media Network (MCSMN) provides training and certification in social media for physicians and is a "global community for those interested in advancing health-related application of social media tools." It seems that you can essentially complete a residency in social media training now if you want to.

Online Information and Social Media Summary

Our participation in social media and other aspects of the digital world in general may have altered the way we behave, interact, and communicate and even process, learn, analyze, and recall information. But how has it changed our relationship with patients, students, residents, and peers? Consider how texting between residents and attendings may have altered the way residents present patients, transfer patients, and learn how to provide care. Think about how the EMR has affected both physicians and patients, from face-to-face communications to age-old doctors' notes about the social and medical histories, physical exams, and treatment plans of their patients. Think about how we access point-of-care information and guidelines with a computer instead of with each other. There is not an area of medical care or medical education untouched by the digital age.

I remember when, several years ago, I first heard medical students or residents presenting information that they said they "found online." I and others would gently but quickly urge them to reference the primary literature: the academic journal or organization where the information originated. Physicians-in-training, as well as physicians-in-practice, need to know how to reference information and to evaluate and question it, especially when it comes to making important clinical decisions. The fear is that, with the abundance of information online with sometimes questionable origins or validity, even physicians may become unfamiliar or unable to discern the authenticity, authorship, transparency, or even the quality of the knowledge they obtain online.

As more physicians use digital tools, additional guidelines become necessary. There is an ever-increasing need for academic leaders, medical organizations, and professional societies to offer institutional support, instruction, standards, and recommendations for online medical information and exchange, regardless of whether physicians are using the Internet to access clinical information, market themselves and their services, inform and educate trainees, communicate with patients, discuss difficult cases with colleagues, monitor employees, provide accurate information and encouragement for patients, or express opinions about the latest healthcare controversies. According to the Massachusetts Medical Society, "Carefully planned and professionally executed participation in social media by physicians is professionally appropriate and can be an effective method to . . . enhance the public profile and reputation of our profession." But we may need more guidelines and support than what is currently provided by medical societies, the American Medication Association, Food and Drug Administration, Federal Communications Commission, and laws like HIPAA to ensure that online medical information is accurate, transparent, and authentic and that personal health information is protected.

At a time when patients expect, if not demand, our digital participation, they continue to search for online medical information and post questions, share experiences, and try to connect with other patients and providers. About six out of ten Americans search for health information online, according to the Pew Research Center.[15] The most accessed online resources for health-related information among the public are as follows: 56% searched WebMD, 31% Wikipedia, and 29% health magazine websites; 17% used Facebook, 15% used YouTube, 13% used a blog or multiple blogs, 12% used patient communities, 6% used Twitter, and 27% used none of the above according to the digital media company Mashable.[6] When the public is asked about their trust in various sources of online information, information from healthcare providers is ranked highest for trust in accuracy. Online information from family and friends and information from local public libraries ranked second and third as "most trustworthy" according to a survey by the Pew Research Center.

Interestingly, 60% of doctors believe that social media improves the quality of care delivered to patients.[16] Increased collaboration among physicians and empowerment and education of the public are some of the hopeful aspects and potential advantages of social media. According to Dr. Eric Topol, cardiologist and digital medicine researcher, access to medical information by patients, at the very least, helps diminish paternalism in the profession.[17] Empowering patients with knowledge is an excellent motive for improving the accuracy and accessibility of online information. But if, in fact, social media has given both patients and physicians more power through new tools and new access, we must hope that it can also improve care somehow through efficiency and responsiveness. That can only occur if we can keep a close eye on who is providing the online information, the accuracy of the information, how digital communications affect us as care providers, and most important, how social media affects the patients we provide care for.

As younger physicians who are more adept with electronic communications replace older physicians who are "non-native" digital communicators, the online world continues to expand into the practice and the profession of medicine. Digital medicine in one form or another appears to be increasingly integrated into our healthcare system. As Swati Bhaskar writes:

> With an increased use of digital medical records, personal virtual assistants, and wearable devices, we expect to see new and innovative ways for physicians and patients to interact through social media in the years to come. As this growth continues, new platforms and apps will develop to facilitate interactions and help more physicians become active social media participants.
>
> —Swati Bhaskar

Of course, new technologies, including digital networks, have the potential to change our communication and our human relationships inside and outside of the hospital. According to Robert Wachter, "part of the work of getting technology to achieve its potential—overcoming the productivity paradox—is to think about these relationships, to be honest about which losses are survivable and which are not, and to build in fixes that recreate (or reimagine) the parts of the exchanges that remain crucial to the work."[18] As more of us (and our patients) become social media users, the playing field of health information exchange, knowledge, and accessibility continues to change—as do our relationships with and care of our patients. We have to remember that, at best, social media enable and encourage conversations. "The expectation is that others will talk back and you will listen," according to Daniel Goldman, in *Bringing the Social Media Revolution to Health Care.*[19]

The problem with online forums of information for security and privacy risks cannot be overstated. Nor can the questionable sources, authorship, conflicts, and motives. But as the information regards symptoms, diagnosis, prevention, treatment, and other medical advice and opinion, we should remember that people's personal information, their health, and their lives are at stake. Whether it is a physician, a patient, or an organization posting, discussing, and imparting information and guidance, there may be large audiences, such as patients and physicians, who are reading and responding. Individuals are potentially making important decisions, such as changing their medical decisions, personal lifestyle choices, and even medication dosages, based on the online information they consume.

Interwoven into any discussion of electronic communications is the problem with the loss of human-to-human connection and personal communications. What happens to our eye-to-eye contact, our empathy and understanding, our healing touch, and other provider–patient connections, all vital to patient care, in this world of online medicine and medical information? As we grasp the realities of the online universe we now live and work in, we are not alone in our fears and our lack of knowledge about the impact of this technology on many aspects of our lives, including our physician–patient interactions. We might benefit from listening to colleagues from other professions for guidance.

Reverend Rebecca Spencer, Senior Minister of the Central Congregational Church in Providence, Rhode Island, can be inundated by the demands of the online world, but she strongly believes in the importance of the ministry of presence. To do this, she says all of us, including ministers and doctors, need time and an absence of computer screens. She remembers that when her husband was dying, they were most helped and moved by the caregivers who listened the best—and that was not always the doctors. But she says small gestures made an enormous impact—small gestures of listening and caring in the clinic were greatly welcomed and appreciated by her and her husband. Digital communication does not allow for human gestures that may touch the heart and heal the soul.

Dealing with the electronic world is not always easy for Baptist Pastor Edward Bolen in Athens, Georgia, who wrote the following:

> My teenage children tell me that Facebook is for old people now; they much prefer Snapchat, Instagram, and Twitter. I'm bombarded with folks who want to connect with me through

LinkedIn or share articles via Reddit or StumbleUpon. The pace of technological innovation and the growing access through portable devices pose a double challenge for clergy.

First, there is the pressure to use an assortment of new communication tools while maintaining proficiency with established skills. Second, there is the stress of finding the time to answer emails, return calls, respond to texts, schedule appointments and visits and reply to Facebook comments. Yet we are being given unprecedented opportunities to reach, share, network and cooperate with members of our congregation and to be part of a growing Christian community beyond the walls of our local congregation. How do we manage these challenges?

—Pastor Edward Bolan

We as physicians face the same challenges—whether its figuring out when to check email, when to finish typing electronic charts, and when we need to turn off our devices altogether. Pastor Bolen's advice may be relevant for all of us bombarded and sometimes baffled by the pervasiveness of electronic communications:

Placing boundaries—even daily limits—on phone calls, email and technology allows for the opportunity to accomplish other tasks and to have a reprieve from the constancy of communication. The disciplines of stopping and organizing are essential skills if we are going to manage productively the information and technology surrounding us.

—Pastor Edward Bolen

There is no doubt that social media changes the way most people communicate and connect with friends, colleagues, and the public. And no one can predict how it will continue to affect patients and physicians. The next iteration of social media and how it might be adapted by those in clinical medicine and medical education or continually affect healthcare, therapeutic relationships, and medical information exchange is anyone's guess.

We know that communicating machine to machine over long distances filled with electrons and without the privacy and intimacy of the exam room is different and fraught with legal, ethical, and professional worries. Social media may be out of our normal professional bounds and often out of our comfort zones because it does not include the bedside discussions with patients or the traditional private interactions with colleagues or professional presentations to academic audiences that we are used to. But this virtual universe of electronic information exchange is a fact of life, and we will continue to wrestle with it for the rest of our lives.

As more "professional" social media options become available, more people appear to be willing to trade their privacy for online global and immediate connectivity. This includes patients and physicians. But are the lessons for improving our communication skills different when we enter this novel medium? It seems that we are discovering this as we learn to ride the daily digital tsunami.

Structure and transparency in social media are often absent, unlike traditional media, where authorship, editing, peer review, disclosure of conflicts of interest, and established protocol and publishing guidelines are still more likely to prevail. While the context, intent, and origins of some social media messaging may be difficult to discern, the public seems to be more on the alert and questioning of social media missives. With the knowledge gained after publicity surrounding scams, hacks, and worse, many now realize that the capabilities and culpabilities of the creators of online information are largely based on the acceptance, interpretation, and ultimate use of the information by the public—or in the world of medicine, on the behavior of patients and physicians.

So how does a centuries-old profession, which still relies on a listening ear and human hands to heal the sick, begin to adopt, adapt, and best utilize digital communications? No one can predict exactly how the electronic age will continue to affect the practice of medicine, the education of physicians, or the health literacy and behavior of the public. As we all ride this virtual highway of electronic data, where billions of others surf, drive, and connect daily, physicians, like everyone else, need to find the best roadmap to help ensure accuracy, accountability, privacy, and reliability both for our patients and for our profession.

Advice for Using Social Media

1. Decide why you should (or should not) use social media professionally and personally.
2. Review the benefits and risks of social media and discuss with trusted colleagues who have experience in this area.
3. Ask your employer, hospital, state board, or professional organization for their social media policy and follow it. (If they do not have one and you have expertise in this area, help them draft one.)
4. Separate personal and professional content online.
5. Do not violate HIPAA laws and reveal any identifiable personal patient information, or else you may face civil, criminal, or professional penalties.
6. Consider taking a course about social media or hiring someone or an organization to help you.
7. Use privacy settings to safeguard personal information and content. (If you don't know how to do this, ask for help.)
8. Routinely monitor your Internet presence and make sure your personal and professional information is accurate and appropriate. You can directly contact and appeal to websites or obtain professional help if necessary to remove negative or inappropriate content.
9. Follow existing professional codes of ethics for physicians when taking part in social media and communicating in online communities. Assume that whatever you write or post can be seen by all—and will be permanent.

10. Pause before posting and think before sending. Protect your patients and their privacy. Protect yourself and your reputation. Always adhere to your professional standards and responsibilities, whatever medium you are using to communicate.

Electronic Medical Records

For many physicians, there may be no greater impact on communications with patients than the EMR. More than 80% of doctors in the United States now use EMRs.[20,21] While much has been written about electronic medical records and their advantages, including quick and reliable access to all clinical information and data, improved legibility and efficiency, ease of locating and sharing information with physicians and patients, graphing trends for patient data, and increased efficiency of communication between different caregivers, the intrusion of a computer into the room where we see patients has been difficult. The disadvantages of EMRs include that it is time-consuming to type in data for some clinicians (systems are sometimes difficult to learn for older doctors), inaccurate information can be pasted into the medical chart, and typing data into the EMR has become a barrier between doctor and patient. There may be no better way to understand the impact of the EMR than to compare old patient charts with new ones: whether in psychiatry or cardiology or orthopedics, the differences are startling. Read a chart from 10 or 20 or more years ago, and you will see how our charting, language, discussions, and recorded medical information have changed. But you may also see that when it comes to information like immunizations, medication allergies, radiology images and demographics, and medical history, we have become attuned to how an electronic system can be advantageous. But like any record, electronic or not, the information is only as good as the person entering it into the record.

How the EMR affects your physician–patient communications is just as important as how it affects the care of your patient. The next time you provide training on your electronic charting program, ask your team how they are making sure that the computer is not interrupting their relationships and care of their patients. The next time that you take a communications training course, ask the teacher for advice on how to limit the negative impacts of the computer on the care of your patient.

How to Prevent the Computer from Interrupting Your Care

- Try to chart outside of the exam room if possible.
- If you must type in front of your patient, limit the time you spend on the computer.
- Make sure the computer is not physically between you and your patient.
- See if you can use a WiFi-connected laptop computer on a mobile high-topped table that you can wheel from room to room while you stand near your patients and push the table away when you don't need it.
- Show the screen to your patient and describe what you are doing.
- Show the patient their information (x-rays or lab results) on the computer.
- Make more eye contact with the patient than with the computer screen.
- During the patient's questions, discussions, and your closure, make sure you are not looking at the computer, and the computer is closed and turned off.

While it is true that in the past, paper charts could be difficult to locate or at times completely lost and sometimes were illegible or incomplete, written medical notes, when done well, were a personal expression of physicians' assessment, diagnosis, and recommendations for the care of their patients. But it is unrealistic in this electronic information age to think that we would ever go back to paper charting. For now, it appears we will just have to continue to think of ways to prevent the EMR from interrupting our communications and care of our patients.

Email: Management, Etiquette, and Professional Guidelines

It used to be that if you had a question or concern for your doctor, you called the doctor's office. You either spoke with a nurse or your doctor to obtain an answer and advice. But more patients want to email or text with their physicians. And more physicians are using email, texting, and other electronic portals to communicate with their patients. At some point email communication between doctors and patients may become as common as telephone calls or even in-person office visits. The benefits of this electronic communication include an efficient exchange of information between visits with your patients. But there are risks, downsides, and specific medical-legal policies regarding email communication that you should know.

With the average person receiving more than one hundred emails per day, the last thing most people, including physicians, need is more emails. However, physicians cite the following advantages of emailing with their patients, as well as using cell phone calls and text messaging: improved relationships with patients; saving time; and better follow-up care. The main disadvantages include misuse by the patient, interference with private life, and lack of reimbursement. Of course, one of the biggest concerns is protecting private health information.

The decision about how, or even if, you are going to use email to communicate with patients may rest solely with you. Your employer, institution, medical society, colleagues, legal advisor, or staff may offer their input, but ultimately the decision will be yours to make. If you do decide to email with patients after reviewing the pros and cons, then you may want to develop a specific set of policies and guidelines to inform both your patients and your staff.

Your written policy regarding electronic communication with patients should include rules that clarify appropriate and inappropriate topics and how best to use email. You may also want to obtain signed agreements by your patients regarding communicating protected health information (PHI) through secure, encrypted, or public unencrypted electronic systems that are not secure. You will want to specify when and how you will respond to emails and make sure your patients have an appropriate understanding and expectations for the role of email communications with you.

Efficient or Overwhelming?

For most professionals, including physicians, email has become a twenty-first-century communication necessity. Invented in the 1960s but with limited technology support until the 1990s, the sheer number of emails produced today illustrates the explosive popularity of constant Internet missives and communiques five decades after the idea was first conceived. Worldwide, some 269 billion emails are sent each day among 3.7 billion email users. The average email user receives more than three thousand emails each month and thirty-six thousand emails every year.

While texting and instant messaging may have an increased presence in our regular electronic communications, for many, if not most, it is traditional email that defines our day and our work as well as our human correspondence. Unfortunately, email clogging up our overwhelmed inboxes can be yet another major obstacle in a sea of electronic distractions that disrupts workflow and decreases productivity for many physicians and others. Email is also an area rife with potential problems for miscommunication, misinterpretation, and missed messages or opportunities. The unforeseeable missteps are many: not seeing or reading an email, not answering quickly enough, making an ill-received attempt at humor, putting an expression in ALL CAPS or with explanation points (that some perceive as yelling), misspelling someone's name, using the wrong greeting or closing, using too many or too few words, and many other false steps.

Learning how to better manage our email communication in all areas of our professional and personal lives can mean improved output and information exchange as well as smoother, more successful lives in general. Of course, the basic rules of good communication do not change with different methods or modes of technology, including email, but additional guideposts need to be established and applied; being professional, courteous, respectful, efficient, and responsive and using common sense should be understood by all. However, the unspoken rules and idiosyncratic behavior of different individuals regarding reading, writing, and sending email seem to have arisen organically as the technology has permeated our world. We have taught each other what we like and dislike but often not without bumps in the road for personal relationships or professional exchanges.

Legal Issues

What some people seem to have forgotten is that emails are permanent, public, and discoverable. Emails can be monitored and recovered. Work or institutional email is not private. Employers are free to monitor these communications as long as there is a valid business purpose for doing so. We have come to understand that personal emails are essentially not private. When legal issues have arisen around email, the courts have ruled in some cases that a search warrant was necessary to recover and retain certain emails, and in other cases search warrants were deemed unnecessary. It appears that institutions, including the government and corporations, can obtain access to our emails and can read, survey, and save them with or without permission in some instances.

According to the American Management Association, more than 50% of companies monitor employee emails, and many of these companies have reprimanded or fired employees for misusing email. Privacy lawsuits regarding email content have exponentially increased in number. Lawsuits arise from emails containing offensive material and often from attempts at making "innocent" jokes that are later deemed racist, sexist, libelous, or defamatory. Email can be admitted as documentary evidence in court, and specific federal and state privacy laws regarding email differ. The courts have sided with the employer or institution accessing a person's email or with the employee whose emails were read, depending on the circumstances.

The First Amendment (freedom of speech) and Fourth Amendment (right to privacy and security of individuals against arbitrary invasions by government officials) to the US Constitution can apply to emails, texts and other electronic communication. In 2010, the US Circuit Court of Appeals sided with an employee saying that government agents violated his Fourth Amendment rights when they accessed his emails without first obtaining a search warrant (United States v. Steven Warshak et al.). The case is notable because it is the first case from the US Circuit Court of Appeals to explicitly hold that there is a reasonable expectation of privacy in the content of emails stored on third-party servers and that the content of email is subject to protection by the Fourth Amendment. However, in a case decided by the US Supreme Court in 2010 (City of Ontario, California v. Quon), the court sided with the employer (a police department taking disciplinary actions against two police officers following an audit of text messages they sent on their pagers that were found to be personal and sexually explicit). The judges ruled that examination of the employee's text messages on a government-issued pager did not violate the Fourth Amendment.

Of interest, where and when the electronic data are stored and who owns the electronic systems holding the data has mostly determined who has legal access to emails and other electronic data. The Stored Communications Act (SCA) of the Electronic Communications Privacy Act of 1986 distinguished between electronic communication services whose only role was to archive and back up transmitted data and systems transmitting or receiving data. Systems or services that actively transmit and receive data can release transmitted data only to the sender or recipient; however, remote services whose only role is to archive or back up transmitted data can release that information to the subscriber regardless of who had sent or received the electronic communication. Of note, in 2018, the CLOUD Act (Clarifying Lawful Overseas Use of Data Act) was passed in the United States. The law contains a provision requiring all email service providers to disclose emails within their "possession, custody or control" when deemed necessary even when those emails are located outside the United States according to Amy Howe writing at scotusblog.com.

Whether you are a politician, public figure, or physician, emails, texts, and other electronic communications are not without risks. Regardless of the nature, context, or ownership of the email, you could be potentially liable. For instance, if what you are writing is determined to be harmful to an employee's or colleague's reputation, it could be considered defamatory in certain situations. Regarding emails, attorney Michelle Fabio writes, "As the age-old saying goes, 'think before you speak' or in today's lingo, think before you send."

Clearly, when it comes to email, knowing that email can be considered a public record if its content contains the transaction of public business and that, legally or illegally, emails can be copied, published, recorded, edited, forwarded, misread, misinterpreted, and misused, as well as appear inadvertently in the wrong recipient's inbox or on the front page of the newspaper, may help reinforce the need for individuals to be careful, cautious, and constitutional regarding these ubiquitous electronic exchanges.

Time Management

One of the biggest downfalls of email seems to be time consumption. Awareness is the first step toward time management of emails. It is important to be aware of your email style and behavior. How often do you check email? How and when do you respond? How often do you delete emails and should you delete them? We all differ, but like all behavior, knowing your own habits and style and learning some professional skills to manage and improve your communication clarity, productivity, vulnerability, and efficiency can be important.

You can decrease your frustration and increase your efficiency by learning how best to utilize your email system.

Organize, Categorize, and Prioritize Your Email

- Organize emails into topics.
- Mark for later action.
- Set up electronic folders.
- Consider setting up separate email accounts.
- Utilize settings to filter out promotions or block spam

You may want to take advantage of different ways to organize emails into topics, mark them for later action, use electronic folders, and consider the pros and cons of having more than one email account. Whether you are someone who doesn't mind having 50,000 emails in your inbox or someone who deletes and organizes emails daily, there are many ways to help you organize and manage the barrage of content and information you now receive daily. It may require knowledge, practice, and time, but like all organizational techniques, it can save time and offer other benefits in the end.

Getting a handle on your email can help determine how productive you, your colleagues, and your staff will be. One method that seems counterintuitive is to set up separate email accounts. This method helps you divide business from personal communications, avoid promotional marketing materials, and be more useful and responsive when handling different activities. Whether you are communicating with colleagues or employees or making reservations, buying insurance, or organizing a family vacation, separate email accounts can help you manage your electronic communications. More than one email account can help you organize different jobs, people, projects, and teams.

Advantages of More than One Email Account

- Separate business from personal communications.
- Organize different jobs, activities, or projects into different email accounts.
- Help avoid promotional marketing materials by using separate email for purchases, reservations, and other online ordering.
- Limit the amount of email to each account.
- Limit the time you have to check each account.
- Set up one exclusive email account (encrypted if possible) for patients.

On average, people today have just less than two email accounts each; some people, of course, have more than two. I spoke with one person who set up a few of his own domains so that in total he had about 40 separate email accounts in the past 15 years. But that is an extreme example—most people have a primary email account they check much more often and one or two other email accounts they check less often. Others might set up one email for their finances or investments, and another for a research paper or specific project they are working on with many other people.

Etiquette and Workflow

Our email communication, from how quickly we respond to exactly how we write and construct our messages, represents our personal style, character, and image we present to the outside world. Similar to our other professional habits, including our appearance, handshake, voice, signature, and attire, email etiquette and responsiveness can be a reflection of not only how we communicate but who we are.

There are ways we can improve the style and efficiency of dealing with this deluge of transmissions.

Advice for Improving Email Efficiency

- Check email only during specific times throughout the day.
- Monitor your time spent on email (be aware and set your own limits).
- Use the delete button daily (delete trash weekly *or* see next bullet).
- Install an automatic archive system if there is any personal, business, or legal reason that you want to save your emails.
- Consider setting up separate email accounts for different parts of your life.
- Create folders (for specific topics or projects).
- Learn how to mark or star for later action or to categorize.
- Learn how to highlight or flag for waiting, reference, or archive.
- Resend to yourself for a date you want to take action.
- Turn off audio or visual alerts (unless you find these helpful and not distracting).
- Advise colleagues on your style and use of email communication (when and how you read and respond as well as what you expect from them).

Emails require various levels of decision-making. Most would agree to open them and deal with or delete them as soon as you can. Author Sally McGhee recommends using "the four Ds for decision-making" instrumental in other areas of our professional lives: deal with it, delete it, delegate it, and/or defer it. This strategy can be particularly beneficial when applied to our daily expanding email inboxes.

The bottom line is that once you set a time to look, open, and read your email, you should have a plan of what you want to do and how to proceed. You should not close an email until you have taken an action and either dealt with, deleted, delegated, or deferred it or put it in a folder, forwarded it, or marked it for future action.

Our communication skills, even in a brief email, are on full and permanent display once we hit the "send" button. Our grammar and syntax, as well as our professionalism and protocol, make an impression on the recipient and reflect back on us whether we realize it or not. The tone of our writing, our attempts at humor, the lack of use of a greeting, the closing or subject line, or a mistaken keystroke, missing word, or sentence may inadvertently be misread and muddle our message and mislead the recipient. Most of us have had at least one or more messages go awry. Reviewing some basic rules to put your best "email foot" forward may help eliminate those.

Advice for Writing Emails

- Use appropriate greetings (e.g., Dear [name], Dear Sir or Madame, Hi there).
- Use appropriate closings (e.g., Sincerely, Warmly, Regards, Thank you, Cheers, Best).
- Be brief (one to two paragraphs at most).
- Refrain from "reply to all" and limit cc/bcc use unless it is necessary.
- Use subject line (update and make accurate).

- Avoid use of **BOLD** or ALL CAPS or all small case.
- Watch tone.
- Be careful with humor.
- Never assume your intent will be automatically understood.
- Check grammar, spelling, and punctuation—be your own editor.
- Spell the recipient's name correctly.
- Check recipient's email address before hitting send.
- Check the accuracy of the subject box.
- Avoid large attachments.
- Read thoroughly first before sending.

Advice for Receiving and Responding to Emails

- Open quickly.
- Respond promptly.
- Confirm receipt.
- Let sender know when they can expect response if not responding right away.
- Never assume the sender's intent of an email you receive.
- Update subject line.
- Avoid hitting "reply to all" unless absolutely necessary.
- Pick up the phone if a more personal, lengthy, or detailed response is needed.

Common Questions

There are some common questions I often hear regarding email. They primarily involve difficult or emotional situations. When the topic of an email is potent or potentially fraught with critical or sensitive material, or the relationship between the sender and the recipient is strained, or their emotions are heightened or conflicted, what is the best way to proceed? After all, not all emails are a simple and quick exchange of information free of emotion, unwritten meaning, or backstory. Email can be easily misinterpreted and cause misunderstandings similar to all communication between humans.

1. **When is it okay to ask to be removed from email lists?**
   If the content is not relevant to you or certainly of interest to you, then it is fine to send out an email request to be removed from an email list. You can ask in a courteous, professional, and succinct way. You can also invite an individual on the list to keep you apprised and notify you if the information becomes relevant to you again or they need you in the future.

2. **When is it okay not to respond to an email?**
   Similar to other areas of your life, using your best judgment can sometimes help you answer your own dilemmas. Why do you not want to respond? How is no response likely to be received? Think back when you sent an email and did not receive a response—if you were expecting one, how did you feel and eventually respond? If an email goes un-answered, then the sender is left to wonder if her email was ever received or if the recipient has another reason for not responding. Depending on the topic, the people involved, and all the different ways you may want to handle it, you can always ask a trusted colleague and look to yourself as the best judge on how to proceed. Waiting 24 hours or more and after a good night's sleep to decide how or when to decide to re-spond to an email can help provide clarity as well. Picking up the phone to respond or seeking out the person for a face-to-face meeting may be the best response of all.

3. **What should I do when sending an emotionally charged email or an email that concerns a very important matter?**
   First, remember that email is not always (or perhaps ever) the best way to communicate. Consider all the other ways

you might communicate best about the issue. If you must send an emotionally charged message by email, type it in Microsoft Word or other word processing application, save it, and then read aloud before you type it, or cut and paste it, into your email to send. You might also first consider sending the email to yourself, then you can see what it feels like to receive, open, and read it as you have written it. If you can, wait a day or two to think about it, then read it once more to yourself before you finally send it.

Exchanging Emails with Patients

What is your current policy with regard to email exchange with patients? What should it be? What are the guidelines from your institution or your medical association? Is it possible to avoid emailing patients when we now live in a world where electronic communication has pervaded all facets of our professional and personal lives? Would it save you and the patient time to utilize email in an efficient, effective, and safe way?

In a survey conducted by Johns Hopkins Bloomberg School of Public Health published in 2016, 37% of patients reported contacting their physicians by email within the last six months, and 18% by Facebook. However, emailing with patients for many physicians still feels awkward at best and unprofessional or even illegal with regard to HIPAA at worst. How do physicians who exchange emails with their patients offer quality communication and care and at the same time protect their patients and themselves from problems?

The following guidelines are from the US Department of Health and Human Services website regarding exchanging emails between physicians and patients:

The Privacy Rule allows covered health care providers to communicate electronically, such as through e-mail, with their patients,
provided they apply reasonable safeguards when doing so. . . .
[T]he Privacy Rule does not prohibit the use of unencrypted e-
mail for treatment-related communications between health care
providers and patients, other safeguards should be applied to reasonably protect privacy, such as limiting the amount or type of
information disclosed through the unencrypted e-mail. In addi-
tion, covered entities will want to ensure that any transmission of
electronic protected health information is in compliance with the
HIPAA Security Rule requirements.
                       —US Department of Health and Human Services[22]

Many would advise that email with patients should only occur over
a protected server that runs behind a firewall, and both sender and
receiver must always be using encryption technology. But your institution or legal advisor may think differently and disagree that
standard email is in compliance with the HIPAA Policy Rule as
long as "reasonable safeguards" are in place.

Of course, using personal email is quite different from using
secure patient portals such as MyChart offered increasingly by
institutions and physicians. But many patients are more familiar
with their own email accounts and often try to use them to communicate directly with their doctors instead of through secure patient portals. (For more information about portals, see section on
Electronic Patient Portals and E-Visits.)

It seems that more patients of all ages want to email with their
doctors for a variety of reasons. Foremost are the convenience and
ease. Getting a quick answer from your doctor by email without
having to make an office visit or leave phone messages is more ap-
pealing for most patients. Nils Bruzelius writes about his experience with emailing his doctors:

Emailing My Doctor: One Patient's Story
by Nils Bruzelius

I am a 71-year-old man who moved from Boston to Washington 17 years ago and have had a variety of experiences communicating with my doctors by email or other electronic means. I have seen several specialists but currently am most often in contact with my primary care provider (PCP) internist and my cardiologist, who have different attitudes toward using email. Their differing ages may have something to do with that, or it may simply reflect different attitudes toward patient privacy and the related legal risks.

My internist is in his mid-60s and shares a practice with one other physician. I have been his patient for about 16 years. He is explicit about not using email but provides some electronic access through a patient portal operated by a medical group. He used to accept and reply to individual electronic messages through that portal, which is cumbersome to use, but he stopped after a couple of years. I don't know why. Now he uses the portal only to provide access to examination and lab results and his comments on them. To his credit, he is very generous with his time during office visits, but if I wish to ask a question at other times, I have to call and leave a message. He does return calls on weekdays, but not on weekends. When I call, the most common response is to ask me to come in to the office, often on the same day.

My cardiologist is in his early 40s and freely accepts and answers emails even on weekends. He is part of a large cardiology practice anchored at a major medical center. I have been his patient since I was diagnosed with nonsymptomatic (except for a fainting spell that led to the initial diagnosis) atrial fibrillation five years ago. I see him roughly every six months, and he has administered stress ultrasounds and carotid ultrasounds over the past two years. Those tests indicate that my coronary arteries are in reasonably good shape.

I am generally open about my medical conditions (including a prostatectomy three years ago) and have no issues that I consider personally embarrassing. I have no need to apply for new health or life insurance, so I have little personal anxiety about medical privacy. I do recognize that it's an important issue. I can't think of a medical problem I would be unwilling to discuss by email except something that indicated I had committed a crime or a sexual indiscretion. Happily, that has not occurred.

I am comfortable researching medical questions on my own with the *Merck Manual* or other print or online resources. However, they are rarely fully satisfying when I'm concerned about a newly developing symptom.

As recently as this spring, I had a reason to want to contact my cardiologist quickly over a weekend. I was in San Francisco, far away from home, when I developed a sharp pain in my upper left chest, a little below the collar bone. I know enough about the symptoms of a heart attack to think that it was probably something else, but I was puzzled and frightened. I had never experienced this kind of severe, unexplained pain in that location. I did not want to visit an emergency department if possible, but I did feel the need for reassurance. I emailed my cardiologist at 10:41 p.m. on a Sunday evening, and he sent a reassuring response at 9 a.m. the next morning. I did not consider trying to contact my internist because, among other things, I knew he would be difficult to reach. As it turned out, the pain receded over the next two days and has not returned. The cardiologist did do a stress ultrasound after I returned home, but it did not find a problem.

I definitely like being able to communicate with my physicians by email because of the timeliness and convenience, and I am careful not to overuse/abuse the access that my cardiologist provides. When the time comes to find a new PCP, I will certainly inquire about email access.

Physicians need to understand their patients' evolving needs regarding electronic communication and try to adapt and be responsive. However, you will want your patients to understand the ground rules for using electronic communication. Obviously, email is not appropriate for emergency symptoms or concerning new signs. Chest pain, signs of a stroke, difficulty breathing, or other alarming symptoms would certainly be issues you would not want your patient emailing you about. Patients need to understand that alarming, complex, or lengthy exchanges may require a phone call, an office visit or a visit to the emergency department. Patients should know that their emails may not be answered quickly but may take several days for the physician or physician's staff to read and to answer. Email messages about nonemergency or noncritical information, as well as concise or simple follow-up questions or inquiries about prescriptions or appointments, may be acceptable to both parties.

You will want to explain to your patients the risks of communicating electronic PHI through any electronic system. You may also want to talk to your employer or your institutional legal advisor about your email system, encryption options, and medical-legal risks as a physician.

Appropriate Use of Patient Email

Potentially appropriate topics for email may include brief clarification about a medication, follow-up visit, lab or x-ray results, nonurgent clinical treatment matters, information about chronic disease management, or appointment reminders. Potentially inappropriate topics range from emergency situations or serious symptoms and any time-sensitive inquiries to sensitive or highly confidential or personal information (e.g., psychiatric symptoms, pregnancy, end-of-life care, life-threatening conditions, HIV status, disability, and legal matters).

Advice for Emailing with Patients

- Email communication requires the same professional standards as all patient communications.
- Gain permission from the patient verbally (put in EMR) or in writing to use email after reviewing potential limitations, including breaches of confidentiality and delays in response.
- Review types of medical communication with the patient that may be appropriate for email and what is not appropriate (e.g., emergencies, private information or personal in nature, lengthy or complex messages).
- Don't use email to discuss a new problem or to relay personal messages to a patient (email is to augment or clarify information from clinic visits).
- Remind patients that all emails exchanges may be at risk for compromising their PHI.
- Remind patients that emails may still require a follow-up phone call or in-person visit.

You can certainly develop a standard form for your patients to read and sign regarding email communication, with information about the appropriate use of email such as prescription refills or questions about appointments, billing, or other nonurgent matters and the limits of security about private health information. You may want to inform them that office staff members may be reading their email and responding if this is true. You may also want to tell patients directly when and how they can expect a response from you or your office when using email.

Electronic Patient Portals and E-Visits

Unlike emails, secure patient portals, such as MyChart, TVR Communications, Sonifi Health, and GetWell Network, are confidential, encrypted, and protected. These types of patient portals are offered by institutions and allow patients a variety of options, including the ability to communicate with their doctor and healthcare team. The sophistication and ease of use vary between systems, but many secure portals allow patients to do a variety of activities, from tracking their health information and test results to gaining access to health education, connecting with providers, and even obtaining advice or medical care for a minor ailment. The portals offer patients the ability not only to exchange secure electronic messages with their providers but also to request appointments and prescription refills, ask simple nonurgent medical questions, read their notes, review follow-up advice, and receive reminders about regular health screening and other activities.

Patients are not always familiar with patient portal systems and often just want to use their personal email or a phone call for the same purposes that are usually provided by institutional system portals. The important difference between personal emails and patient portals are that secure portals are usually encrypted, protected and connected to the patient's medical record.

Patients want easy and quick access to you and their health information, but they don't always know how to do it personally or electronically. Patients may express interest in Web-based tools such as patient portals or other electronic methods to fill prescriptions or track their own lab results, but few are currently doing so. Many patients do not know that their doctor allows for electronic communication or that their hospital or healthcare organization offers patient portals. Some patients have been discouraged by the systems or are intimidated to try to use the portals. Other patients are unwilling to use electronic communication with their doctors even if they are available.

It seems that while electronic communications between patients and physicians are not yet fully developed, accepted, or integrated, it may only be a matter of time before they are. How, when, and why you decide to electronically communicate with your patients will most likely be based on your patients' needs and desires as well as your own knowledge, familiarity, comfort, and institutional support and access to the technology. For primary care doctors, one wonders how many of the 830 million annual office visits per year could be eliminated by electronic communications. The American College of Physicians estimates that 20% of office visits might be eliminated with use of secure electronic communications between patients and physicians.

Patient portal visits or so-called e-visits may increase access to care and reduce the time required for some office visits—or replace some office visits altogether. A recent retrospective study involving chart reviews for nonemergent acute care of adults looked at the nature of care through e-visits and found that 90% of the patients surveyed after an e-visit reported a positive experience and 92% reported that the e-visit had replaced their in-person visit with their doctor.[23] It seems that e-visits may be the next way we take care of patients for nonemergent acute common conditions. But similar to all communications with patients, the more of a relationship the doctor has developed over time with each patient, the more the likelihood that an e-visit for a common ailment will be accepted by both parties and be successful. Of course, e-visits will never replace the intimate, personal, and thoroughness of person-to-person care.

American Medical Association Guidelines for Electronic Communications

The American Medical Association (AMA) has specific guidelines regarding electronic communications between physicians and patients.[24.] According to the AMA, electronic communication can be a useful tool in the practice of medicine but it can raise unique issues especially regarding privacy and confidentiality of sensitive information.[24]

Educating patients on the risks and limitations of electronic communication, obtaining their consent, and allowing patients to decline the use of electronic communications are all outlined in the guidelines.[24]

When physicians engage in electronic communication, they hold the same ethical responsibilities to patients as they do during other clinical encounters. Any method of communication—virtual, telephonic, or in person—should be appropriate to the patient's clinical need and to the information being conveyed.

—American Medical Association Guidelines: Electronic Communication with Patients, Code of Medical Ethics Opinion 2.3.1

Further Reading

Mayo Clinic Social Media Network. https://socialmedia.mayoclinic.org.

Kevin Pho and Susan Gay, *Establishing, Managing, and Protecting Your Online Reputation: A Social Media Guide for Physicians and Medical Practices* (Phoenix, MD: Greenbranch Publishing, 2013).

Eric Topol, *The Patient Will See You Now: The Future of Medicine is in Your Hands*; (New York: Basic Books, 2016).

Sherry Turkle, *Reclaiming Conversation: The Power of Talk in the Digital Age,* Reprint edition (New York: Penguin Books, 2016).

Robert Wachter, *The Digital Doctor: Hope, Hype and Harm at the Dawn of Medicine's Computer Age* (New York: McGraw-Hill Education, 2017).

References

1. Statista, "Percentage of U.S. Population Who Currently Use Any Social Media." Retrieved from: https://www.statista.com/statistics/273476/percentage-of-us-population-with-a-social-network-profile/.
2. Statista, "Most Popular Social Networks Worldwide." Retrieved from: https://www.statista.com/statistics/272014/global-social-networks-ranked-by-number-of-users/.
3. CWC Healthcare, "The Healthcare Social Media Shakeup." Retrieved from: http://www.cdwcommunit.com/resources/infographic/social-media/.

4. ReferralMD, "30 Facts and Statistics on Social Media and Healthcare." Retrieved from: https://getreferralmd.com/2017/01/30-facts-statistics-on-social-media-and-healthcare/.

5. Wisconsin Healthcare Public Relations and Marketing Society. Retrieved from: http://whprms.org.

6. Infographics Archive, "Infographic: Healthcare Industry Building Trust through Social Media." Retrieved from: https://www.infographicsarchive. com/seo-social-media/infographic-healthcare-industry-building-trust-through-social-media/.

7. Social Media Delivered, "Top 10 Hospitals on Facebook." Retrieved from: https://www.socialmediadelivered.com/blog/2015/05/21/top-10-hospitals-on-facebook.

8. L. Campbell, Y. Evans, M. Pumper, and M. A. Moreno, "Social Media Use by Physicians: A Qualitative Study of the New Frontier of Medicine," *BMC Medical Informatics and Decision Making*, 2016;16:91, doi: 10.1186/ s12911-016-0327-y.

9. C. L. Ventola, "Social Media and Health Care Professionals: Benefits, Risks and Best Practices," *Pharmacy and Therapeutics*, 2014;39(7):491–499, 520.

10. S. Bhaskar, "Examining Physician Use of Social Media in 2017," PM360, May 31, 2017. Retrieved from: https://www.pm360online.com/examining-physician-use-of-social-media-in-2017/.

11. I. De Martino et al., "Social Media for Patients: Benefits and Drawbacks," *Current Review of Musculoskeletal Medicine*, 2017;10(1):141–145.

12. N. Pemmaraju, M. A. Thompson, R. A. Mesa, and T. Desai, "Analysis of the Use and Impact of Twitter during American Society of Clinical Oncology Annual Meetings from 2011 to 2016: Focus on Advanced Metrics and User Trends," *Journal of Oncology Practice*, 2017;13 (7):e623–e631, doi: 10.1200/JOP.2017.021634.

13. G. Carbonell, D. B. Meshi, and M. Brand, "The Use of Recommendations on Physician Rating Websites: The Number of Raters Makes the Difference When Adjusting Decisions." *Health Communication*, 2018:1–10.

14. C. J. Donnally III, E. Roth, D. Li, J. A. Maguire et al., "Analysis of Internet Review Site Comments for Spine Surgeons," *Spine*, 2018;43(24):1725–1730.

15. Pew Research Center, "Majority of Adults Look Online for Health Information." Retrieved from: www.pewresearch.org www.pewresearch. org/fact-tank/2013/02/01/majority-of-adults-look-online-for-health-information/.

16. SparkReport, "Infographic: Rising Use of Social and Mobile in Healthcare." Retrieved from: http://thesparkreport.com/infographic-social-mobile-healthcare/.

17. E. Topol, *The Patient Will See You Now: The Future of Medicine Is in Your Hands*, Reprint edition (New York: Basic Books, 2016).

18. R. Wachter, *The Digital Doctor: Hope, Hype and Harm at the Dawn of Medicine's Computer Age* (New York: McGraw-Hill Education, 2017).

19. L. Aase, D. Goldman, M. Gould, J. Noseworthy, and F. Timimi, *Bringing the Social Media Revolution to Health Care* (Rochester, MN: Mayo Clinic Center for Social Media, 2012).

20. Office of the National Coordinator for Health Information Technology, US Department of Health and Human Services. Retrieved from: https://HealthIT.gov and https://dashboard.healthit.gov/quickstats/quickstats.php.

21. B. Monegain, "More than 80 Percent of Docs Use EHRs," *Healthcare IT News*, September 18, 2015. Retrieved from: https://www.healthcareitnews.com/news/more-80-percent-docs-use-ehrs.

22. US Department of Health and Human Services, "Does the HIPAA Privacy Rule Permit Health Care Providers to Use E-mail to Discuss and Health Issues and Treatment with Their Patients? Retrieved from https://www.hhs.gov/hipaa/for-professionals/faq/570/does-hipaa-permit-health-care-providers-to-use-email-to-discuss-health-issues-with-patients/index.html.

23. M. Player, E. O'Bryan, E. Sederstrom, J. Pinckney, and V. Diaz, "Electronic Visits for Common Acute Conditions: Evaluation of a Recently Established Program," *Health Affairs*, 2018;37(12):1931.

24. American Medical Association, "Electronic Communication with Patients, Code of Medical Ethics Opinion 2.3.1." Retrieved from: (https://www.ama-assn.org/delivering-care/ethics/electronic-communication-patients).

3

Public Speaking and
Presentation Skills

We spend a good part of our lives trying desperately to convince ourselves as well as everybody else that we know more than we really do.

—Charles Osgood

There are only two types of speakers in the world, the nervous and the liar.

—Mark Twain

Introduction

As a former television reporter and a current medical educator and practicing medical internist, I have taught many sessions and seminars on public speaking and presentation skills. I have met physicians, clinical researchers, executives, and other health professionals who know that their skills and training in this area are deficient and are very interested in learning how to improve. The good news is that most people are much better at public speaking than they think they are. However, no matter what your current competence level is, you can always do better. After you learn how to identify and tap into your natural personality, attributes, and communication style, you will begin to feel more comfortable.

At some point during your professional life, someone will ask you to give a presentation. You may be honored and elated. But like many people, including many physicians, you may also be nervous and even terrified. There are few activities other than sky-diving, rock climbing, and public speaking that can squeeze your adrenal glands, raise your blood pressure, and cause more of an overwhelming sense of doom than public speaking. In fact, many people will go to great lengths to avoid speaking in front of an audience altogether.

Physicians, throughout their training and careers, are often asked to do a variety of different types of public speaking—from addressing large academic settings and videotaped seminars to speaking in informal informational settings or leading impromptu discussions. Doctors are asked to speak on important clinical topics at hospital grand rounds; discuss preventative health with patients in the community; lecture about their research at a professional conference; talk to medical students or residents at a noon conference; speak to a television reporter about a timely topic; respond at a press conference about a controversial issue; conduct a job interview through video broadcast; Skype with a team of academic researchers from around the world; or conduct themselves on camera for a telemedicine interaction with patients and colleagues.

On September 14, 2018, Dr. Allan Tunkel, Senior Associate Dean for Medical Education at the Warren Alpert Medical School of Brown University, gave the White Coat Address at Cooper Medical School of Rowan University. It was one of the highlights of his professional career. He told the personal story of his near-death experience while suffering from septic shock and pneumonia in the intensive care unit (ICU). He shared important take-home lessons about healthcare for the medical students present that day. The twenty-minute talk was brilliant and well-received by the audience despite the fact that Dean Tunkel committed several errors in public speaking that day. Specifically, he read most of his talk word for word, was hidden behind a podium, and only looked up at the audience occasionally. But Dean Tunkel is a natural storyteller, and what made his talk so effective were his honesty, humor, and true emotion. He tapped into his personal communication style to tell a thoughtful message about his experience.[1]

Examples of Public Speaking Opportunities for Physicians

- Grand rounds lecture
- Community talk to patients
- Professional medical conference presentation
- Noon conference lecture for students or residents
- Television interview
- Press conference appearance
- Video or Skype job interview
- Skype with research team members
- Telemedicine interaction with patients and colleagues

Whether you are asked to speak in one of these varied venues with different media platforms, to different audiences about different topics, or in another type of setting, many of the essential communication skills are the same. Fortunately, they are skills and can be learned, practiced and even perfected. Whatever presentation you give, your communication skills, or lack thereof, will be readily evident to your audience. But you will reduce your anxiety and heighten your performance if you have an increased awareness of your natural skills, knowledge of the mission of your talk, and thorough preparation and practice. I have heard many common misgivings about public speaking.

- "If I could improve one thing about my public speaking, it would be to engage more with my audience. I tend to get very nervous and stick to what I need to say, and I want to get the process over with as quickly as possible. This comes at the cost of not reading the audience or being able to make adjustments and tweaks as needed."

- "Something negative about my public speaking is that if I make one mistake, I struggle to let it go and come back from it. I focus on the mistake that likely nobody else noticed, and it becomes a positive feedback loop of continuing mistakes."
- "Something positive that people have told me is that my pace is good and I seem confident in what I'm saying, which I think is pretty funny because I tend to be nervous in public speaking contexts and not feel confident at all."

Individuals are usually filled with apprehension about speaking in front of a group because they do not realize how good they can be by making minor adjustments and how easy it really is. More often than not, many people will avoid talking in front of a live audience or a video camera if they possibly can. But opportunities to speak are important to take advantage of, whether self-directed or prompted by a request from a superior or an organization. Professional careers and personal connections can be enhanced by giving an outstanding presentation with excellent skills.

I have heard many stories from individuals about avoiding public speaking, from turning down invitations to talk to audiences of patients, to turning down media interviews and even professional opportunities to speak at important conferences. One therapist whom I know declined to be listed on a popular physician referral site simply because she did not want to talk about herself and her work in front of a video camera.

She wrote to me in an email, "I don't like the idea of having to do the video, but that's just me. I am shy."

Unfortunately, medical school, residency, fellowship, and other medical and science graduate trainings offer little if any specific instruction or formal guidance about the topic of presentation skills. Studying science courses, doing well on multiple-choice exams, and memorizing mountains of basic science data may produce knowledgeable doctors and successful researchers but not individuals who are excellent communicators. Although training in this area is changing and more education is becoming available, on the whole there is still little instruction or guidance for healthcare professionals who want to present themselves and their work in the most optimal way.

Whether your goal is to slightly improve your presentation and communication skills or to perfect your performance so that you can become an engaging or even motivational speaker, the rules are the same. Yes, you can become a top-notch communicator and effective speaker. Yes, you should care because if you cannot communicate to an audience about your work, then your knowledge, advice, insight, and opinions will not be heard. And unfortunately, your work may be lost, and your experience and wisdom may never be acknowledged or remembered. Your mission may never get off the ground. The spotlight will shine on others with excellent speaking skills and their work. Those with better presentation skills are often more likely to be promoted, funded and rewarded.

Communication and presentation skills are critical for a successful career. Today, many careers in medicine and throughout the healthcare profession require not only that you give presentations in person to large and small live audiences but also that you are camera-ready and know how to successfully perform in a video presentation or broadcast interview.

> Ninety percent of how well the talk will go is determined before the speaker steps on the platform.
>
> —Somers White

Analyze Your Communication Style

So where should you begin? Unfortunately, the first problem comes with thinking about yourself and your individual communication style. It seems that just thinking about how we speak in front of another person or in front of a group of people, camera, or microphone can cause anxiety. Thinking about our communication is a little like thinking about breathing: all of a sudden something so natural that you have done all of your life becomes awkward and foreign when you focus attention on it or try to analyze it. All of your negative self-damning thoughts, your inner and outer critics, and the memory of individuals in your life who may have put you down, or even your own baseline nervousness, can come back to haunt you and limit your performance.

You may envision yourself as a poor speaker with all of your weaknesses present instead of beginning to see yourself as an articulate and compelling presenter. Knowing your material and the reason you are presenting it and recognizing your skills as a natural communicator are the first steps to helping your performance. Realizing that you have many talents and assets from different aspects of your life and applying those experiences and confidence to your presentations can also be helpful. Just like you have done in other areas of your life, you can apply these inherent human communication and life skills to improving your presentations. Remember that your work and your knowledge are both important. Your audience needs to be informed about your work and what you need to say.

Think about the traits and skills you appreciate in a speaker. Do you like when the person is passionate, clear, understandable, succinct, and comfortable? Would you prefer a presenter who connects with the audience, stays on message, and is able to successfully tell a story or use humor?

Do you appreciate a lecturer who appears to be in charge of the lecture from beginning to end? Are you impressed when the lecturer remains calm and in control no matter what comes up, such as a technical problem with the microphone or a difficult question or comment from the audience?

One truism that may help boost your confidence is the following: remember that, the vast majority of the time, when you are presenting, you will know more about the information than anyone else in the room. There may be some very smart people in the audience, who may ask you some tough questions, but no one knows your presentation and all the information it contains as well as you do. While your audience doesn't know as much as you know about the topic, unfortunately they also may not care as much as you do. Your job is to make them understand the information and make them care about it as much as you do. That is why clear, articulate, engaging, and passionate talks are the most effective and memorable. Make your listeners learn and share your concern and interests. Ensure that the audience hears your message and becomes as passionate and articulate as you are about it.

> If you don't know what you want to achieve in your presentation your audience never will.
>
> —Harvey Diamond

Try to imagine your audience in a positive light. Instead of fearing your audience and imagining a group of enemies, envision the audience as open, accepting, and encouraging. Instead of thinking about the worst-case scenario, imagine yourself giving a great presentation and successfully completing your mission to a group of friends and colleagues. Remember, when you are an audience member, you just want to listen and learn from an informative and accessible presentation. You assume it will go well. Your audience expects you to win, and they are planning for you to give an effective and informative talk.

Another lesson to remember is that practice improves performance. Start accepting opportunities to speak. When asked to do a presentation, don't say no and avoid it. Force yourself to say yes to invitations to give talks. Also, create your own opportunities and talk to your boss or colleagues who might help make these types of opportunities happen for you. The more public speaking you do, to small intimate groups or to large audiences, the better you will become at it. Do not shy away from speaking engagements. Speak more. Each time you present to an audience, it will become easier and you will enjoy it more.

After you have secured a speaking engagement, you will want to do three things: First, remind yourself why you want to speak and create a mission statement for yourself about the goal of your talk. Remember and articulate why you are the best person to give this talk. Second, become an expert about the topic you are speaking on and know your information well. Third, know who your audience is and what they need from you. Realize your inherent worth and, most important, the inherent worth of the knowledge you need to impart in giving an excellent presentation. Transfer your nervousness into productivity; start researching and writing your talk. Also, try to attend a few live lectures or watch some presentations online. Take notes on things you like and don't like. Figure out what kind of presentation skills you want to emulate, then you can begin to gain the knowledge you need to begin to practice and prepare.

> It usually takes me more than three weeks to prepare a good impromptu speech.
>
> —Mark Twain

Even though it is not easy, it is only by focusing on our own communication skills and dissecting them in an objective manner that we can analyze our specific and unique assets and deficits. Then we can begin to learn the important tools to improve. First impressions are key—and that includes first impressions by our audiences about our presentations. Most people make up their minds about us in the first few seconds of meeting us or in the first moments of our lecture; that is why our skills from beginning to end are critical to our success.

There are many common problems people have concerning public speaking. For most of them, there are some easy solutions.

1. **"I've been told I speak too quickly, so I would like to improve this and find a comfortable pace."**
   When most people are nervous, they speak too quickly. Remind yourself that it is almost impossible to speak too slowly. Take a breath. Look out at the audience. Utilize pauses effectively. You should know that while it is hard to speak too slowly, it is possible (and a common error) to speak without enough energy or enough passion. One of the most common errors is speaking too quickly—the other common error is speaking without enthusiasm. Don't commit either of these errors. Try to connect and convince your audience that what you are saying is important. Try to be natural, clear, succinct and make a good impression. Look up at your audience after important points. Have a conversation with them.

2. **"Sometimes I get so nervous when I am speaking that I sort of black out and really lose my self-awareness. I feel like when I am finished, I have no idea how long I have been talking or if I have even effectively gotten my point across."**
   Remember it is not about you. It is about the information you are presenting. If what you have to say is important, then think about how important it is to inform and engage your audience with the content of your presentation. Be organized and engaging. Look out at the audience and build a bridge to them. Make sure they are hearing and understanding your important presentation.

3. **"I don't know about my body language when I am speaking. I try not to fidget, but I hear mixed things about using hands versus not or walking around on stage or not—this is something that I know I do."**
   The more you can focus on your information and the importance of your talk, the more you will be confident and comfortable with your own body language. The more comfortable you are, the more your body language will follow and display confidence. You won't worry about your hands, your

feet, or your body movements; you will use your posture and gestures like you do when you are calm and in control in other situations. (See section on Nonverbal Communication: Our Body Language in Chapter 1.)

4. **"I have been given generally good feedback about my public speaking, but I would say that regardless of external feedback, I tend to feel horrendous while doing it. Some strategies for managing nerves during public speaking would be fabulous. The old 'picture everyone in their underwear' trick doesn't quite do it for me."**

   Instead of thinking of people in their underwear (which I don't recommend), imagine yourself sitting in the audience. What are you expecting from the speaker? You are expecting an informative presentation. You may also be thinking about your next meeting, your daughter's birthday, and maybe even lunch. In other words, the people in the audience are just like you, they have busy lives and just want to hear an interesting and relevant talk—so give them one.

5. **"I feel like I can do okay with thoroughly rehearsed material, but I can stumble a bit if I have to come up with the words as I go."**

   Some people do need to read a script, but instead try to write down bulleted points and know the structure and flow of your talk. You will be able to have a dialogue with your audience instead of reading a script. Just like when you have a conversation with one person, you are not reading a script—think about having a conversation with your audience, only it's one in which you get to do most of the talking. When we "read a script" we tend to lose all of our natural voice qualities and become monotone and emotionless. You will want to give a presentation that is directed to real people in your audience—tell them a story and talk to them as individuals. If you must use a script, mark it up with notes and highlights so you can remember to ad lib, pause and emphasize where necessary. Try to make it more conversational and you will have more success.

6. "I would love to be able to stand in front of others and speak more clearly. I often lose my train of thought and then become roundabout with my word choice."

    Having notes of exact figures or important percentages or other bulleted points in front of you can help you if you lose your train of thought. If you do use a script, you can mark it up so you have notes for yourself. Make your presentation come to life in any way you can. Also, be confident enough that you can easily say, "I think I just got off-track or misspoke; let me back up." Or, "Is that clear to everyone?" or "Are there any questions?"

7. "I wish I could be more succinct and conclude my ideas better rather than trailing off."

    Just like you do when you are speaking to someone else one to one, make your point and then move on to the next point. Put a period at the end of each sentence. Be confident, clear and concise. Each talk should contain between three and six take home lessons. Write these down beforehand. Make sure you discuss all of them and reiterate them before you finish.

8. "I would like to eliminate space-filler words during public speaking. I want to deliver a short speech effectively."

    We all use excess words as crutches or filler words such as "uh," or "yeah" or "do you know what I mean?" and one way to help reduce these is to audio record or video tape yourself. If you hear yourself using unnecessary phrases or filler words as crutches, it will be easier to eliminate them. Catch yourself saying these words in any way you can and work on stopping the use of them.

9. "I would like to have more confidence and focus."

    Think of an activity or hobby you are good at and enjoy, such as golf, tennis, playing an instrument, or another hobby. Transfer your confidence, including body language, tone of voice and other confident mannerisms into your public speaking skills. When you walk onto the tennis court, how confident is your posture? When you play the piano, how peaceful and focused are you? When you are talking to your best friend, how happy and engaged are you? When you are talking to your children, how clear and encouraging are you? Try to emulate these gestures and feelings while speaking to your audience.

10. **"I would like to know how to make eye contact without making it look like I'm intentionally and deliberately trying to make eye contact with people."**

   Look at one face at a time in your audience. Smile and look into people's eyes while you are talking until you see a nod or smile. Pretend the person you see is the only person in the room, then move on to someone else until you gradually build the number of friendly faces you have connected with to as many people as possible in the room. Their facial expressions should calm you down and give you immediate feedback on how you are doing.

11. **"People tell me my voice doesn't sound like it's shaking, but to me it definitely sounds like it's shaking."**

   Take a few slow deep breaths before you begin speaking. This can help calm your nerves and reduce the shaking. You can try to yawn a few times before you walk on stage. Slow yourself, heart rate and ultimately the speed of your talk down. Think of a person, a situation, a geographic location or an activity you love. Close your eyes for a minute and imagine you are in a serene, confident and happy state. Smiling and stretching your body can help as well. Try not to focus on your voice or yourself. Instead focus on the information and how best you are going to engage and teach your audience.

How to Assess Your Public Speaking

If you want to try to assess your own public speaking and presentations, you will need to be open to acknowledging the areas you need to work on. You will also want to listen and learn from others.

1. *Make a list.* Be honest with yourself about your strengths and weaknesses as a communicator and presenter of information, but do not be hypercritical. Write down a list of your perceived strengths in all areas of communication, not just presentation skills and not just when speaking to an audience. Think about your strengths when speaking to a friend or family member or to students, residents, or employees and write these strengths down. Now think about what you would like to improve in your presentation style. You can write down just one word or make a list. Write down any weaknesses you have when communicating or as a presenter. Try to make your strengths a longer list than the list of weaknesses. Next to any weakness, write down the correction you need to make.

   - *I mumble.* I will learn how to improve my articulation and enunciation with specific knowledge, exercises, and practice. (See exercises in this chapter.)
   - *I speak too quickly.* I will learn how to slow down by focusing on serene thoughts and my breathing. I will use pauses and look out at the audience when I speak.
   - *I speak too softly.* I will learn how to breathe properly using a full diaphragm and speak with enough volume, passion, and energy to be heard.
   - *I am afraid to look at the audience.* I will think of other situations where I am confident and can easily make eye contact with others. I will use this tactic as immediate feedback on how I am doing. Reading the facial expressions of my audience is as important as reading the facial expressions while sitting across from someone while having a face-to-face discussion. There is no better and immediate way to realize your audience is confused, bored, or happily engaged, then looking at specific faces in the audience.

- *I am worried about my accent.* There are excellent, dynamic presenters who speak in every language and have many different types of accents and different types of voices. I will embrace myself and my beautiful unique voice and use it to my advantage. If I need professional evaluation or help, I will consult a voice coach or speech therapist. There is usually no reason to eliminate accents that may be different from the native language of your audience.

2. *Ask others.* If you need help making a list of your present communication style, talk to a supportive friend or colleague or even a professional voice coach, speech therapist, boss, or superior to help evaluate how you are at communicating and how you can improve. Ask for your reviews after you give a presentation—and ask your colleagues to tell you honestly how you can improve. You can also ask family members and peers about your communication and presentation skills. Compare this list with the one you created for yourself.

3. *Video yourself.* Finally, record yourself doing a one- to two-minute presentation about your work or topic of interest to you with your computer or your phone. You can use some notes but try not to read a script verbatim if you can help it. Just talk to the camera like you are talking to a friend or a student about your topic. When you are alone, just open your laptop or smart phone, push record, and look into the camera and talk about something you know and are passionate about such as your work, sports, a hobby, or a recent vacation you took. Watch and listen to the presentation. Be kind to yourself. Give yourself an honest assessment. Write down what you like and what you would like to do better. Most people can smile and soften their features at the very least—which, believe it or not, helps their voice sound more natural. Another method to evaluate your voice is to record yourself talking on the phone to a friend or your mother. Listen and evaluate

your natural tone, inflections, speed, and clarity. Most people have wonderful voices when they are talking naturally to friends or family members.

4. *Read your reviews.* When you do give a presentation to a live audience or a videotaped performance for others to watch, welcome any feedback. Look closely at the audience reviews to see where and how you might improve.

5. *Watch the experts.* Watch people you think are good, whether they are professors, politicians, actors, journalists, or even your colleagues. What makes them so good? Try to figure out what it is they are doing that you like. Are they earnest, confident, and making eye-contact? Are they prepared and knowledgeable but also able to handle spontaneous comments or difficult questions? Are their words and their voice clear, pleasant, and understandable?

> Best way to conquer stage fright is to know what you're talking about.
>
> —Michael H. Mescon

Improve Your Voice (Your Instrument)

Your voice is literally your instrument. When you give a presentation, how people feel about your voice will be integral to how they perceive your presentation.

Think about how you react to various types of voices when you hear others presenting. Whether their voices are high and screechy or low and mellow may determine how long you can listen before leaving the lecture or before falling asleep. What about when someone talks too softly? Is that frustrating for you? Or what about when someone speaks indistinctly or incoherently or speaks too quickly or talks too loudly? Is that irritating to you? Besides our body language, our voice quality may have more influence on people's perception of us and understanding of our presentation than any other aspect of our communication skills.

Mistakes People Make with Their Voices

- Pitch too high (screechy)
- Volume too soft (inaudible)
- Energy too low (too mellow or monotone and without passion)
- Poor articulation (mumbling, chewing gum, or fingers in front of mouth)
- Speaking too quickly (it is hard to speak too slowly)
- No pauses (pauses are important and natural)

Do you remember how annoying it can be during a phone conversation with a bad connection or listening to the radio when the signal keeps cutting out? How does it make you feel when the presenter's microphone volume is too loud or too soft? Often, when you give a presentation, you will be speaking through a microphone. It is okay to ask the audience if everyone can hear you—ask specifically whether the volume is too high or too low. You may be speaking perfectly, but if the volume of the microphone is off, or worse yet, if the audio transmission is scratchy or a speaker is broken, your audience may become upset with the sound of your voice and it has nothing to do with you. If the sound system is broken, take off the microphone and speak in a volume that is audible (and pleasant) for the entire audience. You may have to increase your volume.

Always look to your audience for feedback. If even one audience member is wincing or cupping an ear, you know something is wrong. Your audience members will let you know how you are doing. You just need to look at them to see their facial expressions and body language to measure their comfort and understanding of your presentation.

What type of voice is most easily heard and understood? In an article published in *Science Magazine* in 2012, Sabine Louet wrote: "A growing body of evidence from multidisciplinary research in acoustics, engineering, linguistics, phonetics, and psychology suggests that an authoritative, expressive voice really can make a big difference."[2] Someone who speaks slowly with a low voice and a pleasant intonation can be perceived as someone with a commanding influence. According to Louet's article, a good example of an authoritative voice is the voice on the New York subway that says, "stand clear of the closing doors." If you listen closely to professional actors and broadcasters, male and female, as well as different speakers during presentations you attend, you will begin to identify voices you like. Try to figure out what type of voice the person has and what is pleasing, or not pleasing, about it. There are many different voices with different pitches and tones as well as speeds and inflections. The common trait that all successful voices have is that they are authentic and true to the personality of the person speaking. That said, the voice still needs to be supported with a full breath, coming from a confident posture. You need to articulate your important message with the correct volume and energy by properly opening and utilizing your vocal instrument.

Of course, perception of a voice is very subjective. Our culture, geography, gender, age, ethnicity, professional norms, and other biases can influence our perceptions about another person's voice quality. Overall, it seems that low and slow voices from confident male and female speakers using good volume, inflection, and enunciation are often perceived as the most pleasing and commanding.

However, speaking with your natural pitch is just that—it is YOUR pitch produced by not stressing or straining your vocal instrument or trying to imitate someone else. The phrase "speak low" may make some women, and maybe even some men, try to speak lower than their natural pitch. This is a mistake. You should never try to speak higher or lower than your natural pitch. This will strain your body and make your voice sound unnatural, and it can be harmful to your vocal folds. To find your true speaking pitch, say "ho-hummm," and the pitch of the "humming" sound is usually your natural pitch.

Similar to the way a singer determines whether they are a soprano, alto, tenor, or base, you can find and speak in your proper range and comfortable pitch. If you are a soprano, your voice can sound wonderful and melodic unless you try to pretend you are a tenor. Many women in the early years of news broadcasting used to speak with an artificially low pitch, and some still do. But speaking with your natural voice and with your natural pitch will help your voice sound the best. If your throat hurts after giving a speech or at the end of a long day of talking, you may not be speaking at your natural pitch, or you may have other vocal problems that a speech therapist or vocal coach could easily identify.

Listening to a badly tuned voice is like a badly tuned radio.
—Alan Mars, Voice coach

The production of voice, while complex, is still a product of our neuromuscular bodies and can be improved with good instruction and practice. Pitch, volume, timbre, speech rate, and articulation are all essential aspects of our voices and all amenable to training. A speech therapist or vocal coach can help you work on any major problems you may have, such as poor pronunciation, lack of breath control or volume, using the wrong pitch or stuttering. For many people, just practicing a few simple daily exercises and following some specific guidelines when speaking can help improve the quality of their voices. You may also consider taking an acting class, signing up for speech therapy or voice instruction, singing in a chorus, joining a debate club, teaching, coaching, leading groups while hiking or exercise, or engaging in any other pursuits that require you to use your voice regularly, publicly, and effectively.

Almost a decade ago, I joined a chorus. I love music, and I have always wanted to sing. But I also hoped that singing regularly at weekly rehearsals and performing concerts throughout the year would improve my vocal quality and speaking voice so it would remain strong, full, and healthy as I aged. It has worked.

I can prove that regular singing in a group has improved my speaking voice quality by simply watching myself on television or on video. Singing has indeed improved my voice by improving my breathing and use of my diaphragm. The pitch, volume, and modulation of my voice are all more natural now. Just like when you are singing correctly, if you are speaking correctly then your throat should not get tired or sore after giving a talk. When I appear in television presentations now, my voice sounds better at midlife than it did during my twenties when I was reporting regularly on television. Back then, the problems with my voice were numerous. I would run out of air at the end of long sentences. When I was tired, my voice sounded weak, hoarse or artificial. Sometimes my throat would be sore after speaking for long periods of time. But I have learned that relaxing my throat, neck, shoulders, and face and opening my jaw and using my full diaphragm and breath to support my voice (as well as speaking with my natural pitch) have helped eliminate vocal problems.

You may be able to think of many other activities or hobbies, including singing or reciting poetry or storytelling, that require good posture and use of full breaths and vocal muscles to help you regularly produce a pleasant and understandable projection of your best vocal speaking voice. Try to engage in these activities as much as possible. Your voice muscles are like other muscles in your body— you need to use them to keep them in shape. Here are some tips and exercises that can help you improve your voice:

Tips to Improve Your Speaking Voice

1. Speak up and project.
2. Smile when you speak.
3. Slow down and enunciate.
4. Practice deep breathing and controlling your breath on the exhale.
5. Speak naturally and avoid being monotone.
6. Do vocal exercises (listed next).
7. Read aloud in front of a mirror.
8. Record yourself reading and listen to it.
9. Hire a voice coach or see a speech therapist.

Exercises to Improve Your Voice

1. **Good posture.** Stand on two feet in a confident and comfortable manner. Make sure your weight is evenly distributed over both feet. Make sure your feet are hip-width apart. Do not lock your knees. Make sure your feet do not appear nailed into the ground or that you are frozen in position. You can take a few steps one way or the other if you want. Arms at your side. Your posture will affect your voice, and your body language will reinforce your image of confidence. Before we sing, we always stand and spend a few minutes making sure our posture is good. Our hips are over our knees. Our chests are lifted, ribs are in, and abdomen is soft. Move your head from side to side and drop one ear to one shoulder and the other ear to the other shoulder to loosen your neck. Do not stand on your heels or lean on one hip. You should be upright, strong, and supple like a dancer. Do not fidget or be rigid or appear frozen. Stand, breathe, and move with confidence.

2. **Breathe.** Yawn a few times to open the jaw. Now take a deep full breath in on three counts and exhale out on three counts. Now again on five counts in and five counts out. Do this a few times. Diaphragmatic breathing is easy for some and counterintuitive for others. It took years for it to feel natural to me. Singing helped me the most. Put your hand on your belly. When you expand your belly as you breathe in, fill up slowly until you cannot take any more air in; then as you exhale, contract the belly and slowly but steadily breathe out. You will eventually feel the diaphragm literally pulling down and out to fill your lungs with air and then pushing up and inward as you exhale. The expansion as you inhale can be felt around the circumference of the mid-body including the back and the sides. A strong diaphragm and good breath control will give your voice more power and projection.

3. **Relax.** Try to remove any tension from your body, especially from your face, jaw, and neck to your shoulders, back, and legs. Just as tension affects our bodies, it certainly affects our voices. The more at ease you are, the better your voice will sound. You should be alert, engaged, and ready to sing (or give your talk). Do a few shoulder rolls forward and backward. Twist your body gently from side to side. Breathe in and sigh out.

4. **Warm up and strengthen your instrument**. Do some lip trills. This is what you may have called "motor boat" when you were young or playing with young children. Use air to vibrate your lips. You can hum notes or hum a song you know (e.g., "Oh, Say Can You See" or "Happy Birthday"). If you have trouble doing this, gently push or pull the sides of your lips together. You can also try to do a few enunciation exercises as outlined later.

My mother was a professional broadcaster and theater actress. As a little girl, I would ride in the car with her and listen as she practiced elocution and breathing exercises on the way to the broadcast station or theater. She would literally be warming up her vocal instrument so that she would be ready to perform. Try a few of these exercises to help warm up and keep your vocal skills sharp:

Exercises to Improve Enunciation and Elocution

Say these slowly at first and then increase your speed:

- She sells seashells by the seashore.
- How now brown cow.
- Peter piper picked a peck of pickled peppers.
- Red leather, yellow leather.
- Unique New York. Unique New York.
- Betty Botter bought a bit of butter. But the bit of butter Betty Botter bought was bitter. So, Betty Botter bought a better bit of butter.

Read one or two of the exercises daily for at least several days before your presentation. Try to increase your speed. Record yourself. If you memorize a few of these, you will be able to use them as part of your warm-up exercises before you give a presentation.

There are many other exercises to help you awaken and strengthen all of the muscles of the face, tongue, throat, and diaphragm that produce your voice. You can certainly find many of these exercises on YouTube and elsewhere. You can also consider scheduling an appointment with a speech therapist and see if you need any professional help. You can hire a voice or singing coach to help you improve your voice or join a community theater or chorus.

Daily Voice Exercises from Voice Training

1. **Yawn five times.** Soft palate lifts, brings down the lower jaw, and opens and stretches your instrument from the lips to the throat to the diaphragm. Some problems with voice, including a "nasal" quality or even mumbling, can be due to our tongues not being engaged and our soft palates not being lifted. When the back of our throat is opened (like during a yawn), the voice can sound better.

2. **Lip trills.** Awakens and strengthens the muscles around the lips.

3. **Tongue trills.** Engage the tongue, say "butter"; then bend tip of tongue up to roof of mouth and vibrate while making a sound. This awakens and strengthens the tongue.

4. **Say "Ho-hummmmmm" then hum a song or a scale.** With the lips closed and the jaw, mouth, and back of the throat wide as possible. This will open and soften the throat—as well as help you find your natural pitch.

5. **Stifle a laugh.** Keep your lips firmly pressed together. This will activate your jaw, lips, and other face and throat muscles.

6. **Tongue circling in the front of upper and lower teeth.** Both directions. Count 4 right, then 4 left, then 3-3, 2-2, and 1-1. This will help strengthen and improve the agility of the tongue for clearer enunciation.

7. **Say or sing a vowel for as long as you can.** (A) "ah" (E) "eh" (I) "eye" (O) "oh" (U) "oo." Use a full breath. Sing or say one vowel at a time. Open your mouth as wide as you can (look in the mirror) and deepen the back of your mouth and expand your diaphragm.

How can we improve the projection of our voice? When we give a presentation, it is very important that we project to an audience with a full and resonant tone. We need a full breath and the ability to control it to produce this sound. According to Jayne Latz, speech pathologist, our power source is our diaphragm and there are many exercises we can learn to strengthen and engage it.[3,4]

Here are her exercises as well as some I do in singing workshops: Stand or sit up in your chair with your feet firmly planted. (Do not do anything that makes you dizzy or feel sick. If you do feel faint, stop right away.) Make sure you are comfortable. Breathe in and then count loudly as far as you can. "One, two, three, four. . . ." Try it again and see if you can increase the number each time. Make sure during the last few numbers you say that you are still using a strong and full voice. Again, breathe in and then count aloud. Keep adding on to the numbers if you can. Fill your back muscles with air. Count outloud on the outbreath to ten, then to fifteen, and then try to count to twenty loudly and clearly if you can. You can also make a "hissing" sound on the exhale or sing or say a vowel sound ("ah" or "eh"). Look at your watch and time it, and continue to try to make it longer each time. Again, if you feel dizzy or out of breath, stop immediately and sit down.

You can improve your voice by doing these types of exercises daily. After becoming familiar with these types of exercises, you may begin to feel your diaphragm as you take much fuller breaths. Our breath is what produces our voice. The fuller our breath is, and the more we learn to utilize and control it, the better our voices will be. Speaking coaches will work with the specific characteristics of your voice, improving in areas where you may need it the most, from your volume and resonance to enunciation and clarity. There are many tools and techniques that can improve the quality of your voice. But the bottom line is that the better your voice is, the better your presentation will be.

The best thing most speakers can do is optimize their ordinary speaking voice for public performance. Audiences will like you

better for it—and you will feel both more natural and more relaxed as a result.

—Tina Blake, Voice coach[5]

Four Common Mistakes in Presentations

Common Mistakes in Presentations

- Letting your nerves get the best of you
- Reading every word of a script
- Speaking too quickly
- Not engaging the audience

After years of leading communication skills training workshops and programs, I have witnessed many different types
of problems, but there are some common mistakes I see most
people make. Fortunately, there are many relatively quick and
easy solutions.

Letting Your Nerves Get the Best of You

There is no doubt that if you let your mind create a stressful environment, then a shower of negative thoughts and anxiety often
carried by your stress hormones will cascade over you during the
classic fight, flight, or flee response. Once that physiologic mayhem
begins to happen, it is hard to give a calm, clear, and concise presentation. Trust me, even the best public speakers get nervous, but they
stay in charge of their nerves and emotions by doing the following:

1. **Realize it is normal to be nervous.** Expert speakers realize
   that being nervous is a normal response. In other words, if
   you are not nervous, something is wrong. But the level of

nervousness and how you handle those nerves will determine your success.

2. **Channeling nervous energy.** You can channel nervous energy into a good performance with tools such as positive thinking, remembering why you wanted to give this talk and how important the information is for the audience. Remember to use your breathing and visualization techniques. If you are in charge of your emotions, you will be in charge of your presentation.

3. **Think of activities you are good at.** What are you really good at? Think of the professional activities (e.g., operating as a surgeon, speaking with patients or medical students, diagnosing illnesses, talking to employees) or personal hobbies or activities (e.g., golf, tennis, skiing, painting, playing a musical instrument, talking to your children). Now, think about the confidence of your speech and your body language when you are doing those activities. Try to emulate your body language and voice from those activities when you give your presentation. Remember how nervous you were when you were a medical student and you interviewed your first patient? Think of how comfortable and confident you are now when you interview patients and know that you can be the same way in your presentations.

4. **It is not about you.** One way I have calmed down many medical students and residents and improved their presentations of patients' histories and physical exams is to remind them why they are doing the presentation. Presentations on rounds or while handing over care to another doctor are done to ensure that the next doctor or other doctors can take great care of your patient. The presentation is about the patient and not about the student or resident giving the presentation. The same is true for you. Remember, your presentation, regardless of the topic, is about the information you are teaching and

message you are imparting. It is about your ultimate goal and overall mission in doing the presentation; it is not about you.

5. **Visualization and imagery.** I often tell people to imagine that the presentation is over and visualize it playing out in the best possible way. Ask yourself a few important positive questions. How did it go? How great was it? How did you want your presentation to go? How did you want your audience to think about you and remember your information? Now, go out and make your presentation that way, just as great as you imagined it.

No one ever complains about a speech being too short.
—Ira Hayes, US Marine

There is another strategy called a "premortem" (hypothetical opposite of a postmortem) or "prospective hindsight" that business people often use before a project is launched. A project team imagines that a project or organization has failed and then works backward to determine what potentially could lead to the failure of the project or organization. You could certainly do this before giving your presentation. Think about all that you are worried about. Play out each scenario or even write them down. When you review them one by one, they will not look so bad, and you can think of ways to prevent your worst fears from coming true during your presentation.

According to an article in the *Harvard Business Review* written by Gary Klein, "unlike a typical critiquing session, in which project team members are asked what might go wrong, the pre-mortem operates on the assumption that the 'patient' has died, and so asks what did go wrong. . . . The pre-mortem analysis seeks to identify threats and weaknesses via the hypothetical presumption of near-future failure. But if that presumption is incorrect, then the analysis may be identifying threats/weaknesses that are not in fact real.[6]

Here is a sample a pre-mortem you could do before your presentation:

Ask yourself why are you so nervous to give this presentation. Articulate your specific reasons and fears out loud or write them down. Many of your fears may seem ridiculous and somewhat irrational. But you can also begin to create an emergency toolbox if any of your fears begin to come true during the presentation.

- **Are you afraid you are going to freeze and forget what to say?** Bring your cheat sheet of bulleted points and engaging quotes or phrases and, yes, even a script if you must. Prepare and practice beforehand. Take a deep breath. Look out and find a friendly face and smile. Calm down. Go with the flow. Be kind and supportive of yourself before, during, and after the presentation.
- **Are you worried your throat will get dry and you will lose your voice?** Bring water and some throat lozenges and keep them handy. Taking periodic sips of water (not a caffeinated beverage) will keep you hydrated and, most important, will give you and your audience a nice break.
- **Do you fear you will make a mistake or lose your train of thought?** Remember you are human. You might make a mistake. It is okay. Often, your audience will not notice, and even if they do, just apologize and get back on track. Again, bring your specific notes to glance at. Prepare and practice beforehand. Learn to react on your feet. "I am sorry, I think I just misspoke or stated that the wrong way. This is what I meant to say."
- **Are you afraid your audience won't like you or you will look like a fool in front of your peers?** Most audiences want you to succeed, they want to hear and be rewarded with your great presentation. Don't imagine them in any other way. Look out while you are speaking to get immediate feedback from their expressions (and comments or questions) and then adjust as needed.

- **Are you worried you will speak too quickly or in a monotone voice or not be understandable or look too stern?** Videotape yourself practicing the talk. Watch and listen to it, and you will immediately see what you need to fix. Do you need to slow down or smile more or take a few pauses at important points? You may be your worst critic, so you may want to ask a friend to look at the video with you. Once you see yourself, you will likely know how to sound and look better.

- **Think you may faint?** Remember to sit down immediately if you are feeling faint or ill in any way. Tell your audience or others on the panel if you think this very rare event might be occurring.

- **What will you do if you are asked tough questions?** You should always try to predict the questions and comments you might receive from your audience and write down the answers beforehand. Prepare a list of responses such as, "that is a very good question but it is outside of the scope of my talk" or, "that is an interesting and important comment, I am happy to talk to you afterward." Or you can always repeat the question back to them. Ask them to clarify the question and give you more specifics. "That is a good question—why do you ask or what do you think the right answer is?" Answer the question the best you can or simply say, "I am not sure of the answer to that." Many people who ask tough questions just want to be heard and are not attacking you or your work. Even if they are challenging you, it is always best not to react emotionally or become defensive. Remain calm, confident, logical, in charge, and credible. The audience knows you have just received a tough question and, many times, they are just watching to see how you handle yourself and whether you can give an answer. Remember that your audience is not your enemy—they are your students and they are there to learn from you. But you are also there to learn from them, and like any conversation, it is okay to have a good give and take session. Ask them questions.

Learn from them and what they have to say. Maybe someone in the audience knows the answer to the tough question someone else asked—listen to the answer, congratulate them and move on. Create and keep a collegial and supportive environment during your presentation.

- **Could the computer or audio/video equipment fail?** Think about all the possibilities of how technical equipment might fail, assume that it will, and have a backup thumb drive or alternative source of power or microphone or other important backup equipment. Know who and how you can call for assistance and how you might finish your presentation even if the equipment fails.
- **Might the audience boo you or throw tomatoes at you?** Keep a hooded rain jacket handy.

While you should consider the possibility of some of your worst fears happening, generally they will never occur. After you have examined your worst fears about public speaking, begin to focus on the positive aspects of yourself and imagine your presentation being a success. Just like in sports or in theater, visualizing a positive performance while you are preparing your presentation and before you begin are key to an optimal performance.

> It takes one hour of preparation for each minute of presentation time.
>
> —Wayne Burgraff, American philosopher

One major reason that we become so nervous speaking in front of an audience is our fear of being evaluated, assessed, and rejected. Trust me, people are already evaluating, assessing, and, yes, even rejecting you at times, and there is very little you can do about any of it. So, during your talk just be who you are every day. Just prepare and know what you want to say, then practice your presentation, smile, be calm and confident, and remember to imagine and rehearse giving a great talk beforehand.

Visualization versus Premortem

Personally, I like to imagine myself giving a great talk in the exact setting I will be speaking in. I like to close my eyes for a few minutes and actually watch a movie of my performance, similar to what athletes do before they compete. I may even try to visit the location or simulate it in my office. I may record myself with audio or video so that I can watch myself and see if I sound and look okay. The minute I hear and see my recording, I can see things I can improve on. Am I speaking clearly and with enthusiasm? Or am I speaking too slowly or sternly? Am I smiling? Am I pausing and using natural infections? Am I sounding hesitant or unknowing? Am I slowing down and using important pauses when I say something really important? Do I sound natural? Are there any words, names, or data that I am worried about stumbling over? I focus and rehearse and sometimes record these beforehand just to make sure I reduce the risk for error.

Athletes and actors use visualization all of the time. Writing more than two thousand years ago, the famous philosopher and scientist, Aristotle, described the process this way:

> First, have a definite, clear, practical ideal; a goal, an objective. Second, have the necessary means to achieve your ends: wisdom, money, materials, and methods. Third, adjust all your means to that end.
>
> —Aristotle

Creating the mental image of how you want your presentation to go can help you achieve your desired outcome. If you can see it before you perform it, then you can lower the chances of your nervous energy getting the best of you before you speak—and improve your odds of giving a great talk. We must see it before we can believe it.

Before we can believe in a goal, our brains and our bodies have to know what it is going to look and feel like.

Reading Every Word of a Script

There are very few people who can read a speech word for word and make it engaging and effective. Usually, it will sound flat, perfunctory, and unnatural. Most of the people who can read a scripted presentation and sound engaging are actors or professional broadcasters.

But instead of using a script, you should have an outline with prepared bulleted points, data, and conclusions. If you are using slides, this can always help you stay focused and organized. But you still want to include your own impromptu comments, personal stories, or maybe even some light humor. You want to have a conversation with your audience about your key points. If you have a conversation (and don't read a script), you will use natural pauses, modulation, and inflections; you will speak in your normal voice. You will use natural body language and facial expressions. You want to interact and react with your audience. You will not be frozen in a monotone voice or appear like a "deer in the headlights" in front of your audience. The key is to sound like you are having a discussion with your audience. Each audience is different so each time you give your talk it should be slightly different.

If You Must Read a Script

If you must read a script, and sometimes you will, then you need a well-written (and well rehearsed) script in a conversational tone. Use shorter sentences. Write creative, engaging and memorable phrases. Think about cadence and word choice and even poetry or free verse. Mark up your script while rehearsing it. Find the areas where you need to slow down or to pause. Your words need to be powerful, unforgettable, and well-selected. Think about political speeches and remember there is a reason that speech writing is a professional career. When you have a well-written script, you will need plenty of practice to use your natural speaking voice and make your message indelible. Remember to look up and out to your audience as often as possible. You can use your finger or a pen to keep track of where you are so when you look back down you know where to begin again. Professional broadcasters and actors are very good at this because they literally make physical or mental notes about when to look up at the audience and when to pause. (And they rehearse!) It takes practice reading from your notes or a teleprompter to appear natural. If you are using a teleprompter, ask for help beforehand and try to rehearse with the device as many times as you can. If you must read a script, you will have to practice looking relaxed, acknowledging individual faces in your audience, and speaking with varied tone, pitch, and breathing to emphasize important points. You need to allow your audience to listen and enjoy your words. Making notes in the margins of your script to remember to smile, breathe, and make eye contact can be helpful and important. Underlining or highlighting statistics or important phrases can be critical.

Speaking Too Quickly

Many people speak too fast. Most people do not speak too slowly. Again, in reality, for most people it is almost impossible to speak too slowly. The biggest problem with reading or memorizing a script (or being nervous) is that you may tend to speak even more quickly. Reading a script (or memorizing a script) may make you speak too quickly, but even when not reading a script, many people will speak with too much speed. Unfortunately, if you do speak too fast, people will not be able to understand you. Imagine if you spoke a foreign language to your audience. They would not understand, much less remember a thing you said, right? If you speak too quickly, you might as well speak in a foreign language because your audience will not understand you.

By slowing down a speeded-up presentation and using passion and natural inflections and rhythms of your own voice (and making eye contact with your audience), you will be seen, heard, and remembered. Speaking in a flat monotone voice without any energy is not the same as speaking too slowly. In all my years of teaching communication skills, I have seen very few people speak too slowly.

Not Engaging Your Audience

One of the most common problems for many speakers is not smiling, making eye contact, or using natural facial expressions. You need to make eye contact with the audience as much as possible, and avoid a "deer in the headlights" appearance. Smile more and use natural expressions. If you are speaking about a very serious subject, and smiling would be inappropriate, you can soften your facial features and avoid looking stern or nervous by appearing earnest, solemn, calm and encouraging or using other emotional expressions suitable to your topic. Before you begin speaking, take a full breath and look out to your audience. Find at least one friendly face and connect with them. Throughout your presentation, continue to find another friendly face to connect with. If you do this, you will receive three major benefits: First, you will appear calm and confident. People will trust you and look right back in your eyes. Second, you will receive immediate feedback on how you are doing. If your audience is looking perplexed, you are not being clear or believable. If your audience is looking bored or distracted, you are not being conversational, enthusiastic, or engaging. Third, in looking up and out, you will pause, and your speed and delivery will be more natural.

Know Your Mission, Audience, Content, and Yourself

As I mentioned earlier, I developed a lesson to help people improve their public speaking presentations and other communication endeavors. I call it, "MACY" for mission, audience, content, and you. These are the four important aspects to think about before and during your presentation. Before you begin to plan and practice your presentation, try to answer these questions:

- **M—Mission**: What is my mission? Why am I speaking? What is the purpose of this talk? What is my ultimate goal? If I could accomplish one goal with this talk what would it be? State your mission in one sentence.
- **A—Audience**: Who are they? What do they need from me? What do they already know? (You may need to ask them directly.) What do the members of the audience want to know? What will they learn from my talk? How can I be most responsive to their needs?
- **C—Content**: Make sure it is organized and informative. Use words and phrases that make your message concise, relevant, and engaging. Tell a story if you can. Overall, make sure your talk has a beginning, a middle, and an end. Be prepared with specific points you want to make but also be prepared to improvise. Have a conversation with your audience about your important points. Do not read every word from a prepared lecture.
- **Y—You**: Be prepared, organized, and rested. Be calm, clear, and confident. Rehearse the entire talk at least twice in the week leading up to the talk. Know why you are the best person to give this talk on this day. And remember, it is not about you—it is about the information you are presenting.

I am convinced that most people have all the tools they need to be a great communicator. To help you improve, it usually requires identifying and tapping into your natural communication skills and then using them in an unnatural setting. It also requires identifying and eliminating obstacles or habits that may be getting in your way of giving a great presentation.

How can you identify and tap into your natural communication style and skills? Think about when you are with friends, trusted colleagues, or beloved family members. Stop and listen to yourself when you are talking to a friend or doing an activity that you are good at. Most likely you are clear and confident. You know you have something to say and something to do, and you go about doing just that in a natural way. Your body language and posture, as well as your facial expressions and your voice, tell everyone you know what you are doing. That character and persona is what you need to tap into to transfer these attributes to your presentation skills. But how do you translate being poised, eloquent, fluent, effective, persuasive, lucid, expressive, intelligible, comprehensible, and understandable into another setting—particularly at a podium in front of a large audience or in front of a video camera in a television studio?

First, we need to tap into the basics of what makes a good communicator. Again we can turn to Aristotle and the 3 critical elements of a great communicator he identified. Ethos is our character, credibility, reputation, trustworthiness, tone and style. Pathos is our emotional imaginative impact—the stories we tell to make a personal connection. Logos is the reasoning, arguments, facts, figures and case studies we use—the logic and the actual words we speak.

We do all of these naturally when we are engaging in an activity we are good at. Do you remember the first time you played the piano, examined a patient, performed surgery, or followed a recipe? My guess is that you were not as confident and capable as you are now doing those activities, right? How did you gain that confidence?

Yes, with knowledge, expertise and practice, but also focusing not on yourself but on the task at hand. You need to play the music on the piano keys, not think about yourself playing each note. You need to examine that patient and present your findings to your team and not focus on your words or pauses or posture. You need to swing that golf club or tennis racquet for a successful game and not think about how nervous you are trying to perfectly connect with the ball.

You need to focus on the task at hand. You need to play the concerto and win the point. You need to give a great presentation. The information you are presenting needs to be communicated. The audience wants to hear your message and learn from you. Communicate with confidence and by using your natural abilities and talents.

Observe Natural Communicators—including Yourself

Try to study people who are natural communicators. When you are listening to a live lecture or watching a TED talk or a news broadcaster on television, think about what qualities you appreciate in a speaker. What makes them effective at communicating? What is their body language? What are their facial expressions? How lively and interesting is their voice? How are they connecting with the audience or the camera? How do they make you feel as if they are talking directly to you? Do you think they are nervous? Trust me, they are, but they are letting their message be more important than their nerves.

Most important, you need to observe and study yourself. Again, what do you sound and look like when you are with your best friends or family? When you are talking to your children or sailing your boat or riding your bike? When you are engaging in familiar activities in familiar settings, what does your voice sound like? You can transfer this confidence, conversational speaking style, calmness, and clarity to your public speaking.

Imagine that Your Audience (or the Camera) Is Your Best Friend

Think of someone who makes you feel both calm and confident—someone who believes in you. Bring that person to mind and really see and hear them. They are looking and listening to you, and they want not only to hear what you have to say but also for you to do a good job. Whether this is your best friend, a trusted colleague, or a family member, imagine this person is in the audience (or in the camera) and then speak directly to him or her.

One Skill You Would Like to Improve

If you could improve one aspect of your presentation skills, what would it be? Most people usually know where they need to improve their communication capabilities.

Do you speak too quickly? Do you try to memorize and end up sounding like a machine speaking in a monotone voice? Are you too nervous to make eye contact with the audience? Are you so uptight that you do not blink or smile or use your natural facial expressions? Do you forget to take a big breath and calm yourself beforehand? Can you be calm and focused and just have a conversation so that you incorporate pauses and natural inflections in your speech? Can you improvise or react when you get a tough question or something goes wrong with the equipment? Write down your important points and answers to tough questions you may be asked before you begin.

Again, the most important tip I can give is to be yourself and have a conversation with your audience.

Avoid the Standard Format if You Can

Many medical talks, like published abstracts, academic writing, research articles, and patient notes (e.g., histories and physical exams) often follow a standard format. Most medical presentations use or misuse slide programs such as PowerPoint. But that doesn't mean you have to—especially when speaking to a nonacademic audience. Even in an academic setting, think about ways to break the mold and be more effective and informative, and your audience will thank you.

How can you improve your clinical talk, academic research, or other important presentation to your peers?

Why should you avoid jargon even when speaking to your peers? In every profession, including medicine, we use jargon and acronyms assuming everyone in the audience understands us. The problem is that it is not always true. Often, using professional jargon, buzz words or acronyms becomes a bad habit and a crutch that limits the discussion instead of broadening it. Many times, you and your peers have either never known or have forgotten what the real meaning is. And even if that is not true, there is nothing that makes a talk flat and uninspiring as one that is riddled with idioms and professional vernacular. Challenge yourself, with your writing and your speaking, to avoid the use of jargon, abstruse professional terminology, and acronyms. Try to stop using words like "stakeholders" "big data" "population health management" and "innovative care strategies" and just use words to explain exactly what you are talking about. Pretend you are talking to someone outside of health care. Use plain English. If you must use acronyms (and medicine is filled with them), at least say the whole phrase or name—at least once say endoscopic retrograde cholangiopancratography instead of ERCP or lateral collateral ligament instead of LCL. You will not only broaden your audience (not everyone always knows the professional jargon you may use), but your audience will listen more closely and maybe even learn and or remember something they had forgotten.

Do you and your audience really know the meaning of all the acronyms you use? Even if you and they do, what is the harm in saying the full meaning once in your talk? Words are powerful and informative. Acronyms are slang crutches and shortcuts that can become outdated or misleading. They can clutter our presentations, preventing us from fully engaging our brains. I challenge you to avoid any use of acronyms the next time you give a presentation.

Slide Presentations: PowerPoint and Others

The vast majority of presentations today still utilize Microsoft PowerPoint, but there are certainly other slide presentation programs now available, including Google Slides, Prezi, Visme, Haiku Deck, Emaze, Keynote, Projeqt, Slidedog, Slidebean, and Zoho Show. Slide-building software programs are invaluable tools to help illustrate and illuminate your information. Unfortunately, many people make major errors in using the programs. First, most people use too many words on each slide. Many speakers fill each slide with text or even write out their entire talk on each slide. Then they proceed to read whole paragraphs and even sections of chapters or expect their audience to read large sections of text from each slide. This is not only inefficient but also boring and frustrating.

You want to use PowerPoint or another slide program to elucidate and augment your talk not as a crutch or a distraction. Illustrations, graphs, photographs, formulas, data points, life cycles, and other simple but efficacious graphics should bring your presentation to life. They should be simple and easily understood. You should use as little text as possible. You also should not overwhelm your audience with moving graphics or too many bells and whistles. You are giving a lecture, not putting on a circus of multimedia examples. Think of yourself as an audience member. You want to be informed and enlightened, not befuddled and bombarded with special effects.

The slides should speak for themselves. You should not have to "read" your slides to your audience. You can refer to them or let them illustrate what you are saying but do not read them outloud. You want to make eye contact as much as possible while talking to your audience. You are having a conversation with your audience and making important points. Slides should illustrate information clearly and memorably than your spoken words. Again, do not write out your talk on your slides to use as a crutch. Know your talk well from your rehearsals and then illustrate the important points with graphic slides.

[S]cientists look toward the projected slides a lot when they present. As a result, they fail to maintain eye contact with the audience, which is a very important part of a good presentation. In my study I found that, during a 20-minute presentation, speakers turn toward the projection an average of 3 times per minute.
—Brigitte Hertz, PhD, Wageningen University, Netherlands[7]

Best Practices for Slide Presentations

- Write the outline of your talk before making any slides.
- Limit the number of words on each slide.
- Slides should augment your information (not distract).
- Use graphs, illustrations, formulas, and pictures.
- Important visual message on each slide should speak for itself.
- Use 10 relevant slides for twenty-minute talk (or 20 slides for forty-minute talk).
- Slides should communicate something you cannot say in words.

Informal Audiences: Patients and the Public

If you have the opportunity to speak to a group of patients or members of the public or others in a community or academic setting, by all means do it. Some physicians are more intimidated talking to a group of nonphysicians than they are speaking to peers, but they shouldn't be.

Talking to a group of patients or members of the public is no different than talking to patients one to one or members of the public one to one. True, these are not medical colleagues, and you may need to speak in simpler terms and explain technical points or complex medical information, but you should be doing that regardless of your audience. With a nonmedical audience, you should think about talking to individual members of the audience, not a large group of faceless audience members. Think about talking to specific family members and friends who are do not work in medicine. You can still be informative and engaging even without using scientific, academic or professional words or jargon.

Fred Sullivan Jr. is a professional actor who teaches public speaking. He teaches his students to imagine they are throwing a ball to the audience when they are speaking, and the audience has to catch it and throw it back. This image illustrates the dialogue you have to have with your audience—you need to make sure they are hearing and understanding you. Take your cues from their facial expressions, ask them questions, and encourage their questions to make sure you are throwing the ball (your information and message) and they are catching it (understanding your message and responding to your information).

Tips for Excellent Presentations

- Make eye contact with specific audience members.
- Relax—be comfortable and confident.
- Tell a story (beginning, middle, and end).

- Use humor (but be appropriate and be cautious not to offend).
- Ask the audience questions.
- Poll your audience by asking for a "show of hands."
- Encourage the audience to ask you questions.

The most precious things in speech are the pauses.

—Sir Ralph Richardson, actor

In 1986, I read *The Man Who Mistook His Wife for a Hat* by the brilliant Dr. Oliver Sacks. I learned that he was speaking at the Harvard Graduate School of Education that fall and I could not wait to attend. I arrived early and noticed Dr. Sacks in the hallway outside the classroom by himself. I approached him with my pen and my copy of his book in hand. But when he noticed me, he snapped at me with a menacing look. I don't remember exactly what he said, but I quickly went into the classroom and took my seat near the front. Throughout his lecture, I noticed he was sweating profusely. Many of his slides (shown through an old carousel slide projector) were out of order. He seemed frustrated. Even though his lecture was not as smooth as I thought it could be, it was still interesting. But I was embarrassed and nervous myself about approaching him again. The minute Dr. Sacks finished, and once the applause and cordial exchanges ended, he came directly over to me and apologized. He explained how nervous he was about public speaking. He asked to sign my book. I still have the book and cherish his autograph to this day. But it was an early lesson that even some of the finest minds (and writers) among us are not always naturally great lecturers.

Of course, in the decades that followed, Dr. Sacks became a public figure and gave many interviews and talks and often appeared on television. He clearly became more comfortable speaking to groups, and perhaps he received some professional communications training along the way. But he certainly improved his skills and hopefully reduced his anxiety.

Don't Be Afraid to Ask the Audience Questions

Peggy Noonan, author and political speech writer for President Ronald Reagan, spoke at Harvard Kennedy School in the late 1980s. I squeezed into the standing-room-only auditorium packed with students, faculty, and others. After being introduced, the accomplished and brilliant Noonan went up to the microphone and looked out over the audience. The room was silent. No one could wait to hear from the person who wrote some of the best political speeches of our time, including President Reagan's "Boys of Pointe du Hoc" speech on the 40th anniversary of D-Day and his address to the nation after the Challenger explosion, and Vice President George H. W. Bush's famous phrases "a kinder, gentler nation" and "a thousand points of light."

She stood at the microphone, looked out over the audience, and said, "tell me what questions you have." My heart sank, when I realized this phenomenal speech writer had not prepared her own speech for us. I was a little taken aback. But then Noonan proceeded to take an hour of questions from the audience and gave the most eloquent, thorough, and informative answers you can imagine. She gave the audience exactly what they had come for—a chance to ask their specific questions. There was a standing ovation from the audience at the end of her talk.

While I don't recommend you doing what Noonan did for your presentations, I do think the take-home lesson is to try to give the audience what they want and need from you. Know your audience. Know what they already know and what they need from you. Keep looking directly at their faces during your talk to see how you are doing. Encourage comments and feedback. Leave time for questions either throughout the talk or at the end.

What is difficult about speaking to a group of nonpeers is that you may not know what they already know and what they hope to learn from you. Whether you are speaking to a group of patients at the community library or legislators at the state capitol, here are some tips that can help you "read" your audience:

1. **Ask the audience questions.** Start out by asking a few questions that would help you understand their level of understanding. "Does anyone know the year AIDS was first described?" "Can anyone tell me what country has higher overall vaccination rates—Cuba or the United States?" Asking a question is a great way to begin your talk—and your conversation with your audience. Of course, you should also try to figure out what burning questions your audience hopes you will answer in your talk. Go ahead and ask them a few open-end questions before you start. You can answer their questions right then or better yet write them down and tell them you will make sure you address those questions in your talk. Some audience members will just want to make a comment and not have a specific question. You can always respond to comments and expand on them. "That is a very good point and here is some more information about that topic" or "I will talk more about that later in my talk" or simply "That is interesting" and then move on.

2. **Introductions.** Ask for a few volunteers from the audience to introduce themselves and tell you what they are hoping to learn from your talk. If there is time, and it is a small audience, you can certainly have everyone introduce themselves.

3. **Encourage comments.** Before you begin, tell your audience that you welcome questions and comments either throughout your talk or at the end. It will help you and your audience warm up and get to know each other if you take questions early on. After you begin your presentation, you can decide whether you want to be interrupted during your talk. I usually

prefer to be interrupted throughout my talk because then my presentation becomes more of a conversation with the audience. But you can also tell your audience that you will leave enough time for questions, answers, and discussion at the end of your talk, which may help you keep from getting off point or running out of time. If you do this, then encourage your audience to write down any questions and make sure to ask them when you are finished with your talk.

But what if your audience is a camera? Here are some lessons about giving a presentation on a television broadcast or via a recorded video.

Video Skills: On-Camera Presentations

If you are speaking to a camera, first of all you need to do two things: (1) forget the camera is a camera, and (2) imagine the lens is your best friend. Again, imagine that someone who helps you feel calm and confident (a family member, colleague, or a friend) is literally sitting inside the lens. Talk to that person.

If you can actually imagine that your best friend, beloved family member, or trusted colleague is inside that lens, then you will lean into the camera and talk to them directly. Your body and your voice will be more natural. Of course, there is no one looking back at you giving you immediate feedback, as with a live audience, but imaging that someone you admire is listening to you will help you look into the lens and be a sincere, effectual and natural communicator. Your eyes should not be reading a script or darting around the room. You should be smiling and pausing and using your natural compelling and useful facial expressions. Everyone looks better when they smile, breathe, and let their body and their breath follow their thoughts and the mission of communicating important information.

Like an actor, if your mind can think of a person you trust and like (or even love) and who helps make you feel comfortable and confident, then your body, face, and voice will ease, and you will be on your way to using your own best style to communicate authentically.

If you are speaking to a camera, you need to make "natural" eye contact with the lens. This can be intimidating at first. But if you can imagine that the lens is the actual face of your best friend or trusted colleague, you will look and speak naturally. If you can imagine that a family member or friend is literally inside the lens, you won't appear stone faced or have a "deer in the headlights" look. You don't want to grimace, squint, or think about how much or how little you blink or if your smile is okay. You don't want your eyes to look like they are reading a script or darting around the room and making you look shifty. If you can look straight into the camera and just truly imagine talking to the friendly person you have identified, then you will loosen up and appear less formal. You will be on your way to using your own best style to communicate authentically, even when speaking to a camera.

Writing for Video

When you write down the actual message and information you would like to say to the audience (through the camera), the information needs to be clear, concise, and conversational. Usually, you will want to state your name and your title first. Just like you would in person, introduce yourself and tell the audience the title of your talk. You should tell them what they are about to hear and why they should listen. Introduce yourself and grab their attention. You will want to tell a story to keep your audience engaged. Use short sentences. Use meaningful memorable phrases. Do not use jargon or professional buzzwords. Make sure you have written down five important points you want to make. Write down any statistics or data you need to cite, but present all of this information as a story and in a conversational style. Make the words sound as if you are talking to your best friend. Make it passionate and informative.

Name It and Give It a Title

You will also want to give your talk a brief, memorable, and descriptive title. After the audience hears a title, they are ready to grasp the details and explanation. When we give something a name or a title, we give it meaning so that we can make it tangible and memorable. We help our audience know what to expect with a title.

Delivery

Be yourself. It is not about you. It is about the information. Breathe. Smile. Look the person (or the camera) directly in the eye. Watch others and see what works—but more important, watch yourself when you are talking to your friend or family member about something you are excited about. Slow down in important sections. Pause after an important point. Don't speed up or throw away lines (your name, title, project). Sit up or stand. Be enthusiastic and passionate. Make them care about what you are saying.

Camera and Technical Skills

Framing. Try to make sure that your head, shoulders, and upper torso fill two thirds of the video screen. Try to make sure there are no windows or mirrors or ceilings in the picture. Sometimes you will see a very nice interview done in front of a window—but usually the lighting is perfect, and there are trees, sunshine, and a pretty landscape seen through the window. This is difficult to make look professional and usually requires professional photographers and lighting specialists.

Lighting. Most video cameras, even those in our computer screens or phones, make automatic adjustments as needed for lighting. You usually do not have to worry about doing any special lighting yourself. Usually the best lighting is natural lighting from windows nearby (but the windows should not be seen in the frame). If you must use the lights in the room (or on the camera), make sure that when you take a sample video, your face is not too dark and the overall lighting of the room is pleasing and not distracting by being too bright or too dark.

Clean office and neat background. Make sure your office, desk, bookshelves, and room seen in the video are clean and neat. You do not want a distracted or cluttered background. You want the exam room, office, or desk area to appear organized and professional. It should not be obtrusive. You can first take a still frame shot of yourself as you will appear in the video and then look at it and make sure it looks as good as it can before you begin videotaping. Make sure there is not an overflowing trash can or several piles of paper or clutter nearby.

Your appearance. Dressing in professional business attire is usually recommended. You want to be comfortable but make sure that what you wear is conveying the image you want to project. You should wear whatever you would wear in person to speak to the audience for whom you are videotaping. Follow whatever is the professional norm in your environment. Remember that it is usually better to be slightly overdressed than underdressed. Your clothes and your appearance are your image.

Clothes for On-Camera Appearance

- Professional business attire is usually best.
- Wear something that fits and is comfortable while standing or sitting.
- Avoid wearing black or very dark clothing.

- Avoid all white (usually includes a doctor's white coat); white doesn't look good on camera.
- Avoid busy, loud, or small prints.
- Avoid large jewelry because it can cause noise.
- Have a suit, shirt, or dress lapel or collar to clip a microphone on.
- Do not wear hats or large earrings.
- Wear dress shoes (assume your legs and feet will be seen).
- For men, navy blue suits with light shirt and tie look best on camera.
- Women can usually wear pastels or bright solid colors.
- Bring a backup suit or dress in another color in case you need to change.

In preparation for your presentation, think about the following: Your words. Your voice. Your body language. Your authenticity. Remember to just try to have a conversation with your audience. Do not read your speech or use a teleprompter. Smile. Breathe. Focus. Educate and engage your audience and they will remember you and the information you taught them.

Tips to Improve Vocal Skills and Presentations

- Do more presentations and public speaking (not fewer).
- Watch and study the experts, TED talks, lectures, political speeches, and other presentations.
- Practice and record yourself giving a talk (find others to join you).
- Listen (or watch) your recording and see what you need to change. Do you need to speak slower or pick up the pace? Be more animated? Smile more? Be more relaxed?
- Take an acting class or public speaking seminar.
- Find a voice coach or public speaking teacher.

- Consult a speech therapist.
- Join a chorus (singing can improve breathing and voice quality).

Practice, Practice, Practice

Always practice. Do a run through with another person if possible. But at the very least, read it out loud at least once. Time yourself. Try to videotape yourself. This can be very helpful.

Advice for Video Presentations

- Your head, shoulders, and upper torso should fill up two thirds of the video screen. You should be the largest object in the picture.
- The background should not be distracting. It should be clean and professional. Take a still picture first with you in it just the way you will be sitting when you talk to the camera, before you start. Make sure you and your background look the way you want them to.
- Make sure you are eye to eye with the lens. You do not want to be looking down at or up into the lens.
- Do not sit in front of a window or a mirror when videotaping yourself.
- Make sure a lamp, plant, or other object does not appear to be growing out of your head. Background objects should be to the side of you generally.
- You should be well-lit and well-framed.
- Have a conversation with the lens as if your best friend were sitting inside the camera.

- Think about standing because it will give your voice and body more energy.
- If you sit, sit up comfortably with good posture.
- Do not look frozen or assume a "deer in the headlights" look.
- Soften your features and smile more.
- Be confident that you know the information you are presenting.
- Don't think it has to be perfect. Speak naturally. Just talk and have a conversation with the lens. Talk like you do in your everyday life. It is okay to have a few filler words and not speak in complete sentences.
- Make it a great video presentation!

Advice for Live Presentations

- Relax, lean into the microphone or podium, and first say hello and introduce yourself.
- Make sure you have water nearby.
- Remember to ask the audience questions about their background and their experiences, including whether they are comfortable with the room audio, visuals, lighting, and temperature.
- Talk to the audience like it is an audience of close colleagues and friends.
- Speak in your natural voice with inflections and enthusiasm.
- Wear professional attire that you are comfortable wearing while sitting or standing—and that projects your desired image.
- Make sure there is a place on your clothing to attach a microphone if necessary (suit jacket or collar lapel).

- Do not read a script. Memorize or write down the important points you want to make and the flow of your talk, then just have a conversation about your topic.
- Create a catchy and memorable title for your project.
- Know your opening and closing lines and make them memorable.
- Use pauses effectively before or after you state important points.
- Uses pauses to look out at your audience.
- Speak slowly and clearly but with good energy and passion.
- Do not look frozen or fearful.
- Soften your features and smile more.
- Think about standing because it will give your voice and body more energy.
- If you sit, sit up comfortably with good posture.
- Have a great presentation!

Further Reading

Matt Abrahams, "A Big Data Approach to Public Speaking," *Stanford Business,* April 4, 2016. Retrieved from: https://www.gsb.stanford.edu/insights/big-data-approach-public-speaking.

Dorie Clark, "A Checklist for More Persuasive Presentations," *Harvard Business Review,* October 11, 2016. Retrieved from: https://hbr.org/2016/10/a-checklist-for-more-persuasive-presentations.

Peggy Noonan, *On Speaking Well: How to Give a Speech with Style, Substance and Clarity* (New York: Regan Books, 1999).

Steve Olenski, "Five Communications Skills that Make Good Leaders Great," *Forbes,* March 29, 2016. Retrieved from: https://www.forbes.com/sites/steveolenski/2016/03/29/five-communication-skills-that-make-good-leaders-great/#48bbe0457ae9.

Charles Osgood, *Osgood on Speaking: How to Think on Your Feet without Falling on Your Face* (New York: William Morrow, 1988).

William Safire, *Lend Me Your Ears: Great Speeches in History,* Updated and expanded edition (New York: W. W. Norton, 2004).

Rebecca Shambaugh, "To Sound Like a Leader, Think about What You Say and How and When You Say It," *Harvard Business Review,* October 31, 2017.

Retrieved from: https://hbr.org/2017/10/to-sound-like-a-leader-think-about-what-you-say-and-how-and-when-you-say-it.

Allison Shapira, "Breathing Is the Key to Persuasive Public Speaking," *Harvard Business Review,* June 30, 2015. Retrieved from: https://hbr.org/2015/06/breathing-is-the-key-to-persuasive-public-speaking.

References

1. A. Tunkel, "White Coat Address at Cooper Medical School of Rowan University," September 14, 2018. Retrieved from: http://cmsru.rowan.edu/students/whitecoat/.

2. S. Louet, "Your Voice: Your Passport to Authority," *Science,* January 27, 2012. Retrieved from: https://www.sciencemag.org/careers/2012/01/your-voice-your-passport-authority.

3. J. Latz, *Communicating Up the Corporate Ladder* (Oceanside, CA: Indie Books International, 2016).

4. J. Latz, "Be Clear, Concise and Confident with Corporate Speech Solutions," *YouTube,* January 30, 2017. Retrieved from: https://www.youtube.com/watch?v=8rQiqC6q5gUJayneLatz; https://www.corporatespeechsolutions.com.

5. T. Blake. Retrieved from: http://www.tinablake.com/category/voice/.

6. G. Klein, "Performing a Project Premortem," *Harvard Business Review,* September 2007. Retrieved from: https://hbr.org/2007/09/performing-a-project-premortem.

7. Hertz, B., Kerkhof, P., and van Woerkum, C. "PowerPoint Slides as Speaking Notes: The Influence of Speaking Anxiety on the Use of Text on Slides," *Business and Professional Communication Quarterly,* 2016;79(3):348–359, doi: 10.1177/2329490615620416.

4

Traditional Media

Introduction

I have worked for many years as a medical journalist. In fact, I was a medical journalist before I became a physician. In my work, I interviewed countless numbers of clinicians and research scientists and translated hundreds of medical articles and ideas. I worked with many medical writers and editors at newspapers, magazines, medical journals, television and radio news organizations, and the Internet. I taught students and physicians about journalism and communications. As a member of medical journalism organizations, I have worked with medical journalists and communications experts. I have studied the impact of the press on physicians and have written articles on medical journalism during editorial fellowships at the Kaiser Family Foundation, the *New England Journal of Medicine*, and Harvard School of Public Health.

I believe there are several reasons that physicians should understand the media and consider engaging and working with the press.

As a physician you may have no interest in talking to, or engaging with, the press. You might consider news coverage of medicine and health topics superficial, sensationalized, or misleading. Or you may be a physician who is interviewed by reporters regularly on your area of expertise; one who avidly reads medical articles in newspapers and magazines; or a physician who writes her own newspaper column or hosts a medical podcast or television show.

Regardless of your experience with and opinions about the media, improving your understanding of reporters' roles, responsibilities, and professional guidelines may help reduce your anxiety and potentially help you relate to journalists and use the press. Most physicians spend years talking to patients before anyone from the press asks them to do a media interview. Interestingly enough, the ability to speak to patients can translate to doing well with the media, and vice versa. There are similar skills involved in talking with patients and reporters: listening and understanding their questions and concerns; explaining complex issues in brief, clear, and accurate statements; and making your key points logical, comprehensible, and engaging. At some point in their career, a few physicians may decide to write an op-ed article, a news or magazine article, or a book for the lay public. But why do this? Because as a physician, you have access to important knowledge as well as a perspective and a point of view valuable to the public. You have something to say and something to teach the public because you do it every day in your practice and your profession.

Reasons to Engage with the Media as a Physician

1. The press influences the public, government officials, and key stakeholders in medicine, research, and healthcare policy.
2. The press informs your patients and influences their perceptions, expectations, and decisions.
3. Talking to reporters may help you talk to your patients.
4. Your patients may ask you questions regarding medical news articles.
5. Your role as public health educator can be expanded by the media.

6. Your knowledge, skills, opinions, and research can be disseminated to a broader audience by the media.

7. You may learn something from the media, from research ideas and clinical issues to topics outside your expertise and changes in public health policy.

But before you decide to interact with the media, you may want to familiarize yourself with guidelines from various organizations including the American Medical Association (AMA). In 2017, the AMA adopted a list of guidelines for ethical physician conduct in the media. In the report, they recognized that the knowledge and skills of physicians represented in the media can greatly benefit the community as a whole. However, the opinions that informed the guidelines were cautious and warned that the expectations of physicians as members of the medical profession and persons in the media are not always compatible.[1]

"Physicians involved in the media environment should be aware of their ethical obligations to patients, the public, and the medical profession," according to the AMA. The association reminds physicians that their "conduct can affect their medical colleagues, other health professionals, as well as the institutions with which they are affiliated." The guidelines emphasize many different topics including the importance of physicians protecting patient's privacy and confidentiality, disclosing all conflicts of interest, encouraging the audience to seek out qualified medical care, and to only speak on topics related to their expertise. Of course, as physicians involved in the media we must always "uphold the values, norms, and integrity of the medical profession."[1]

Traditional Media

Traditional media is defined as all forms of mass media that have been around since before digital technology became available.

Think about the newspapers, magazines, television and radio news programs, and other journalistic institutions and publications that existed before you owned a smart phone or an email account. It is true that most, if not all, traditional media now have an online presence, from websites, Facebook, and Twitter to blogs and online streaming forums, so it is sometimes hard to tell the difference between traditional media and social media. Yet, there is a great difference. Most newspapers, magazines, and broadcast news entities are still considered traditional media and follow the same journalistic standards and ethics of the journalism profession. Examples include your local newspaper, radio or television news as well as the *New York Times, PBS News Hour, ABC World News Tonight, Fox News, NPR, Time, Newsweek,* the *New Yorker* magazine, and others. The press is often referred to as the "fourth estate" and is protected by the First Amendment to the US Constitution. Like other professions, journalism enjoys academic programs for training, professional credentialing, institutional guidelines, and national conferences and awards such as the Pulitzer Prize and Peabody Awards. All of us, including those who work in medicine, benefit from our freedom of speech and our freedom of the press. The press publishes information and opinion on a variety of subjects in the United States and other countries, including issues regarding medicine, science, and public health. But the current landscape of journalism is under stress from financial, structural, and electronic changes underfoot. The future of the profession is often difficult to envision and even medical journalism has undergone major sea changes since its inception.

Medical and health coverage in the news media became popular several decades ago, when a national newswire writer first began writing for the lay public about clinical and research articles published in the *New England Journal of Medicine* in the early 1970s. Shortly thereafter, many newspapers and television news programs began to develop regular health sections or reports on medicine and science. On November 14, 1978, the *New York Times* began publishing *Science Times,* a weekly newspaper section about health and science. Other major news outlets quickly followed and created health beats with their own medical reporters. Before that time, there was only sporadic news coverage of medicine in the lay press. It seemed that physicians and journalists wanted little to do with each other. Today, medicine is a popular topic; it seems that no research finding or issue in medicine or healthcare story goes unexplored by the media. Journalists, including physician journalists, seem to translate, illustrate, and expose the complexity, mystery, and insularity of medicine on a daily basis. How the media frames and explains medical topics has a substantial impact on the public and perhaps even the profession and practice of medicine. On any given day, the news media may influence patients and physicians as well as the direction of research, funding, guidelines, and government regulations.

As physicians, part of our job has always included public health education and advocacy. Many physicians and scientists are notable, in part for the books or articles they have written for the public, from Hippocrates (460 AD to 370 AD) and Maimonides (1135–1204), to Lewis Thomas (1913–1993), Sherwin Nuland (1930–2014), Oliver Sacks (1933–2015), and Richard Selzer (1928–2016). Current physician writers and journalists include Jerome Groopman, Atul Gawande, Siddhartha Mukherjee, Abraham Verghese, Sherry Fink, Perri Klass, Danielle Ofri, Abigail Zugar, and Lawrence Altman to name just a few. Journalism, like medicine, began as a public service. Today, physicians increasingly view medical journalism, like they do their own profession, as a public service and as a way to inform the public and educate their patients.

Impact of Traditional Media on Patients and Physicians

But what about the impact of the news media on physicians and patients today? When I was a fellow at the *New England Journal of Medicine* in 2003, I conducted a national survey of 408 physicians assessing their perceptions and attitudes about the impact of medical news reports on clinicians, patients, and healthcare delivery. With the vast and constant stream of health news and medical information to the public, I was curious about how the news media and specifically how medical information in the popular press potentially affected the interactions between physicians and their patients. (In my survey, the definition of "news media" or "popular press" referred to television and radio news programs, newspapers, magazines, and the Internet and did not include advertising such as commercials or print ads.)

The results of my survey revealed that most clinicians perceived medical news reports as significantly affecting patients and physicians as well as their interactions with each other in a clinical setting. The majority of respondents believed that news media was a major source of health education for patients and reported patients often asking them about information from news reports. And yet, most doctors felt that the quality of medical news reports was only "fair" and gave the media a grade of "C" for quality of medical information.

Survey of Physicians on the Impact of Medical News

- 39% of physicians reported feeling "uncomfortable" when patients inquire about medical news in the media.
- 59% of respondents graded the quality of medical news reports as "C" or "fair."
- 62% of surveyed physicians reported first learning about medical developments in the popular press before another source such as a medical journal, meeting, or lecture.
- 75% of physicians believed the news media is a MAJOR source of medical information and health education for patients.
- 86% of physicians reported patients inquiring about information from news stories "very often," "often," or "sometimes."

- 90% of physicians believed that health news reports lead to unnecessary tests, workups, medications, or therapies.
- 95% of physicians indicated the popular press present medical information in a way that is out of context, misleading, or exaggerated "very often," "somewhat often," or "occasionally."

Although I completed that survey several years ago, little has changed except perhaps a broadening of the reach of the news media through the Internet. The news media continue to be a major source of health information for patients and a common source of medical information for the public and leaders in health care.[2,3] There is a reason that the *Journal of the American Medical Association*, the *New England Journal of Medicine*, the Mayo Clinic, and the Centers for Disease Control and Prevention, along with most other major medical institutions and publications across the country, continue to send press releases and other notifications to the lay press. It is difficult to know exactly to what extent medical news reports and medical journalism affect our world and our patients' worlds, but it is clear that the perception of influence is significant. So, if your patients are getting their information, particularly clinical information, from what they read in the newspaper or see on television, you and other physicians and researchers should at the very least be aware of the content of medical news and, if possible, become involved with the press in some capacity.

Understandably, many physicians, as well as research scientists, are reluctant to engage with the media either because they don't know how or are fearful of such an engagement. In a study from 2014, researchers found that even though scientists were reluctant to engage in public communication at the expense of academic productivity, there were important reasons to consider communicating with the public through the press, including improving a "scholar's scientific impact."

[O]ur survey of highly cited U.S. nano-scientists, paired with data on their social media use, shows that public communication, such as interactions with reporters and being mentioned on Twitter, can contribute to a scholar's scientific impact. Most importantly, being mentioned on Twitter amplifies the effect of interactions with journalists and other non-scientists on the scholar's scientific impact.[4]

Why Should You Talk to the Press?

An important component of a physician's duties is that of a public health educator; there may be no better way to educate a large segment of the public than through the media. Award-winning medical journalist Roger Sergel, now Editor-at-Large for SurvivorNet, worked for many years as the ABC News senior medical producer and editor. He spoke to my class at the Warren Alpert Medical School of Brown University about medical journalism in November 2017. His lecture was based, in part, on a query he sent to doctors across the country with the question, "Does talking to the media help you talk to your patients?" The responses he received and relayed to me outside of the course were from leading physicians who often interact with the media. Many had important lessons to share.

One key aspect I have come away from is the journalistic approach to a story is the exact opposite of how we docs approach it. You in journalism have the headline first, then the key points, then some context and at the very end, details on the methods. We [in medicine and science] give the background, then methods, then slowly walk through results, and THEN we give the punchline of what is new and some context on why this is important. So, in talking with journalists, I have to train my head to pick out in one clear sentence, what our five-year study found—the simple key finding. Then try to briefly put in some context and also give high level methods to show how we found it. That has been the key for me. Focusing on the important stuff.

—Dr. Christopher P. Cannon, Senior Physician, Brigham and Women's Hospital Professor of Medicine, Harvard Medical School

Talking to the press . . . really does help convey important messages to patients without the use of medical jargon.

—Dr. Deepak Bhatt, Executive Director of Interventional Cardiovascular Programs, Professor of Medicine, Harvard Medical School

I think the principles of talking effectively with patients and reporters are the same and that the key is listening WHILE you talk so that you can ascertain whether the patient (or the reporter) is fully grasping the conversation. Just as with patients, I might explain a particular situation to a reporter at different levels based on the questions that come back to me as the discussion moves on.

—Robert T. Schooley, MD, Professor of Medicine, UC San Diego Health Jacobs Medical Center

Another advantage of engaging with the press and talking to reporters is that you may benefit from learning new information that both the public and your patients are interested in. You may also be intrigued and inspired by reporters' questions. In my years of interviewing physicians and clinical researchers, I had more than one tell me that they gained new ideas for their research based on the questions I asked or the discussions we had during my interview.

I can say that many of my research ideas and studies had their origins from questions from the media.

—Dr. Lori J. Mosca, Columbia University Medical Center

Whether you are talking to reporters one to one or speaking at a press conference, the more you speak to reporters, the more you will hone your communications skills and be able to engage and educate different audiences.

I believe that speaking with the press is important, as a public service and an opportunity to inform and educate the public about often complex or confusing medical information. . . . Physicians and surgeons who have acquired the communication and interpersonal skills to effectively inform the media about complex medical matters are equally successful when communicating with their patients and families.

—Dr. Timothy J. Gardner, Christiana Care Health System

When you decide to talk to the press, using common language and clear, simple, accurate explanations can help reporters and the public understand complex topics. Your performance will improve with preparation. After reviewing the information and updating yourself on the important specifics of the topic, you can help by writing down brief messages that encapsulate the information with an appropriate level of information, context, and emotion. Think of the way you explain things to patients. You do not give a lecture with all of the background information, data, research findings, exceptions, and caveats. You just need to explain the topic and answer their questions in an informative and succinct way. There are many rhetorical devices that can help your communication, including use of a story, repeating engaging words or phrases, use of alliteration, and the art of first telling the listener what you are going to say and then making a clear summation. Sometimes the use of metaphors, analogies, and similes can be helpful in creating images and trying to distill and explain information. We will look to the *Oxford English Dictionary* to help us remember the difference between each of them.

Metaphor: a figure of speech in which a word or phrase is applied to an object or action to which it is not literally applicable. A metaphor is a figure of speech containing an implied comparison. Here is one example you might use in medicine: "We have made great advances in medicine with gene mapping." When we speak of gene maps and gene mapping, we are using a cartographic metaphor.

Analogy: a comparison between one thing and another, typically for the purpose of explanation or clarification. An analogy is a similarity between like features of two different things. An analogy is comparable to a metaphor and simile in that it shows how two different things are similar, but it is more of a logical argument. For example: "The human heart and a pump." "An analogy between the workings of nature and those of human societies." "The brain and a neurologic switchboard of connections."

Simile: a direct comparison between two different things in order to create a new meaning; it usually begins with "as" or "like." For example: "Life is like a box of chocolates." "Diabetes coats red blood cells with sugar like a baker coats glazed donuts with sugar." "White blood cells are like biologic soldiers protecting us from pathogens."

Healthcare professionals use metaphors and similes often. Phrases like "biological clock," "thunderclap headache," and "orphan drug" can be helpful when communicating with journalists as well. Of course, military metaphors and other controversial metaphors from "war on cancer" to "doctor's orders" or the "patient is losing the battle" are pervasive in medicine, and many have rightly pointed out that they are unfortunate and often unnecessary.[5] We need to be mindful of the words we use and how they affect the meaning of what we are saying—whether we are talking to reporters, the public, or patients. We want our words to provide clarity not confusion.

The language and interpersonal tools you have used all your life, whether communicating to friends, family, students, or your patients, will be the same tools you will want to use when talking to the media. One thing to remember is that you should know more than the reporters do about the topic or they would not be interviewing you. You may be considered an authority on the subject or at least a well-informed professional. Be open, honest, clear, and informative. Stick to your own area of expertise. Don't say anything that you do not believe to be true and do not violate any professional codes of ethics, including the Health Insurance Portability and Accountability Act (HIPAA). Listen to the reporter's questions and try to answer them as succinctly as possible. Don't prattle on or give too many details. Try to answer their questions in one to three sentences then stop and see if they understood. Make sure you are making eye contact and be aware of your body language. Watch the reporters' facial expressions to see if they are understanding you. If you can find out more about the story they are working on and what they need from you (as well as who else they may be interviewing), then you can provide the right information. Try to make it more of a conversation. Remember, you can first ask the reporters some questions to assess their understanding and awareness of the issues. After you start the interview, you can always ask them if your explanations are clear and if they have any other questions before the interview ends. Always make yourself available for follow-up questions through email or phone calls. Often, when I am writing an article, I will inevitably have a few follow-up questions after the interview. The information and clarifying statements in follow-up interactions are often the most important to me—and the information and quotes that I end up using in my articles.

Advice for Talking to the Media

1. Prepare brief specific points to focus on.
2. Stay on topics in your area of expertise.
3. Distill your message into factual and engaging sound bites.
4. Be succinct, informative, and accurate.
5. Provide the information with context and the right level of details.
6. Explain why the information is important.
7. Don't get bogged down in complex background, details, or caveats.
8. Use metaphors, analogies, and similes where appropriate.
9. Use simple words—break the information down into component parts.
10. Avoid jargon, acronyms, professional buzzwords and medical-ese.
11. Don't be provoked or become emotional.
12. Be honest.
13. Stay in control, on point, and on message.
14. Be available for follow-up questions by email, phone, or in person.

Many organizations, from the American Medical Association to the American Association for the Advancement of Science, offer help in communicating with the press. Professional organizations and media specialty associations offer workshops and resources for helping physicians and researchers interact with the media. Your employer, hospital, or state medical association may have communications specialists or training centers or individuals available to help answer your questions.

Getting a Call from a Journalist

A friend related a story of a physician who received a call from a television reporter about an injury affecting a professional sports player. The physician was not caring for the injured player, but he was aware of and understood the injury. The problem came when the physician was so nervous when the television reporter was interviewing him that he became tongue-tied and was unable to communicate a simple explanation of the orthopedic injury and the prescribed treatment. The reporter was unable to use any of the interview, and unfortunately the doctor's "sound bites" were never aired in the television report.

If you want to be a source for journalists, expect to be contacted at inconvenient times. If an outbreak of an infectious disease occurs or a famous person is diagnosed with a disease or suffers a particular injury, reporters will contact physicians who can help explain the issues.

This often places physicians in an awkward position not only because they are not used to talking in "sound bites" for reporters but also because they may not know the specifics of the case or the accuracy of the reports in the media about the news story. When President Barack Obama had a skin tag removed, or presidential candidate Hilary Clinton fainted, or famous television personality Anthony Bourdain committed suicide, reporters called doctors for explanations. Of course, you will always want to preface your comments with clear reminders that you are not commenting specifically on the famous patient who is not under your care, but you can talk generally about the medical condition and try to answer their questions.

Whether you are an expert on a particular clinical ailment or you happen to be a well-spoken emergency department physician during flu season or when there is another medical issue in the news, you may someday be contacted by a journalist who would like to interview you. If you want to be the one who is contacted, then you need to let the communications or public relations (PR) expert at your hospital know that. The PR specialists are always in touch with the media. They usually know the journalists personally and know how to get in touch with them. You can also contact reporters directly. Let them know that you are an expert in certain fields and would be happy to talk to them if an issue in your area ever arises.

So, what should you do when a reporter contacts you for an interview? First, don't panic. You can always call your PR person at your institution or hospital, if you have one, to get immediate help and advice. You will want to find out as much as you can before you agree to an interview, including asking the journalists who they work for, what they need from you, and what their deadline is. Try to find out as much as you can about the story they are trying to write. If you already know the reporters and have worked with them before, this process will be much easier.

Usually, the reporter will have several basic questions about one topic, such as the flu or sunburns or a medical issue in the news. The questions will usually not be difficult, and if you can remain calm and just give brief, understandable, and informative answers, it will be a good experience.

> My ability to simplify and explain to my patients from the perspective and concerns that are important to them, has led me to be able to speak with reporters more clearly!
>
> —Diane Harper, MD

> By having to focus a response in a "sound bite," it helps to develop a concise way to present an overview to patients (and then we can drill down further if they wish and/or it is appropriate).
>
> —Darrell Rigel, MD

> At the CDC [Centers for Disease Control and Prevention], we used to say "our patients are the public."
>
> —Andrew T. Pavia, MD

Issues to Consider before Agreeing to an Interview

1. Ask for help from a media or public relations person.
2. Find out the name of the journalists and who they write or report for.
3. Find out as much as you can about the story they are writing and specifically what they need from you.
4. Review their past work if you can. Do an online search of their work by name or news organization. Search "site:[newsoutlet.com][name of reporter or key words of topic].
5. Is the reporter a print, television, radio, or online reporter? Will you appear on camera or will you be interviewed over the phone? Do you have to go to a broadcast station or will they come to you?
6. What is their deadline? (If they need you today, you may not have time.)
7. Who else are they interviewing? What are their sources of information?
8. Remember it is okay to decline an interview.
9. Consider recording the interview.
10. Ask to talk "off the record" first if you want to find out more about what they need and do not want to be quoted.
11. Assume everything you say is "on the record" unless you state or ask otherwise.

If a journalist calls you and you do agree to be interviewed, you can always ask the journalist to send questions to you beforehand. Some will do this, while others will not. But one way or another, by talking first through your institution's PR specialist or talking by phone directly with the reporter, you should be able to find out about the story the reporter is pursuing and what type of information the reporter may need. After you have vetted the journalist and you feel comfortable with the topic, then you will want some tips on reducing your nerves, staying in control, and making it a good experience.

Advice for Talking to a Journalist

1. Know the issue—do your homework.
2. Prepare for the interview by reviewing what you want to say.
3. Be able to break down the topic in component parts.
4. Prepare a few sound bites (one-sentence statements). Practice beforehand with a friend or colleague.
5. Record your sound bites and listen back to them.
6. Explain concepts in one or two sentences.
7. Talk to reporters like you talk to patients or family members.
8. Be truthful, sincere, and succinct.
9. Make it understandable, memorable, and engaging.
10. Teach them why the topic is important and relevant.
11. Continue to return to your main key points throughout the interview.

Once you have completed the interview, you can ask to see your quotes before the story is published. This is more work for the reporter, and I don't always advise it if you have worked with the reporter before but if you feel the need to do this, then just let the reporter know. It is not out of bounds to ask to see your quotes before the article is published. Just tell the reporter that you would like to see your quotes to make sure what you said was clear; the reporter can then either email or call you before the article goes to print. Of course, this is harder to do in a television interview, but not impossible—the reporter or producer can email you your sound bite or play the audio of your sound bite over the phone for you. This can be a good way to clarify what you said and to know what quotes they will use before you see it in print or watch it on television. You cannot change the quotes, but you can ask to give more context or background. You can also say you misspoke and would like to provide a new quote to use. But if your quotes are accurate, don't split hairs and try to change them, which is just more work for the journalist. Often, people I have interviewed will want to sound more authoritative; remove slang, common words, or filler words; or try to add information to their quotes. This is usually not necessary and is much more work for the journalist. Quotes are supposed to be conversational and add a human voice to the reporter's story. Quotes are not supposed to be long complex scientific sentences or prepared statements that sound artificial.

You can always record the interview with your own phone or recording device so that you have an audio copy of what you said and the context of the entire interview for your own records. This is not necessary but is not a bad idea in case there is any dispute about what was said. Talk to your communication specialist about this. Be forewarned that wanting to record the interview may alarm the reporter, especially if the reporter just wanted to ask you a few questions about flu shots or how to prevent frostbite or dehydration. If you begin making all sorts of requests, recording the interview on your own, and acting like it is some kind of *60 Minutes* investigative interview, then it may cause a problem. Always just use your best judgment when it comes to being interviewed by a reporter. Remember that you can always ask for help and guidance from a PR person, legal expert or colleagues at your institution.

Using Caution when Talking to the Media

Public relations experts advise everyone to proceed with caution when talking to the media. There is a reason that "public relations" is a profession. PR people specialize in dealing with reporters and the media. Their full-time job is managing the images and messages of individuals and institutions as well as trying to train and prepare people to deal with the media. They can be enormously helpful in managing your dealings with the press. But eventually you may get a call from a reporter, and you may or may not have a PR person to help you—and then what should you do?

Try to be responsive. Don't ignore a reporters' calls or delay your response. Find out who they are and what they want from you. You can always have your secretary or assistant help you with this. When you do talk to the reporter, understand whether you are "off the record" (nothing you say can be used in their article) or "on background" (what you are saying can be used by the reporter but not attributed to you by name) or "on the record" (your quotes and information will be used and attributed to you). You can also always ask for advice from a lawyer or other professional advisor.

When you are interviewed, make sure you have prepared your bullet points but by no means read a script. Be conversational. Imagine you are talking to one of your patients. Relax and make eye contact. Obviously, don't lie, exaggerate, say something you do not want broadcasted, or breach HIPAA regulations by sharing any identifiable personal patient information.

What happens if the reporter tries to provoke you? Or asks questions you were not prepared for? You need to stay in control and not get emotional. Much like communicating with an angry patient, you will want to keep control of your emotions and remain calm. You can stop the interview by just saying, "We need to stop here. Thank you." You can then calmly and politely excuse yourself.

Most interviews are not "gotcha" investigative interviews. If you are worried about such an interview, then by all means, hire a PR specialist and an attorney. Most interviews with doctors are about the latest cholesterol guidelines, new health recommendations, or the latest nutrition trends. If you are responsive, knowledgeable and prepared, tell the truth, and understand the rules of engagement, then speaking to the press can be a good experience in your role as a public health educator.

Before Talking to a Reporter

- Ask for help from a PR person, communications specialist, or an attorney.
- Be prepared.
- Keep it simple.
- Predict the questions the reporter might ask.
- Memorize bullet point answers. Don't bring a script.
- Prepare your important points as sound bites.
- Use metaphors and analogies.
- Have a conversation with the reporter.
- Imagine talking to one of your patients or students.
- Relax and make eye contract.
- Don't breach HIPAA regulations or share personal information.
- Don't assume anything is off the record—make your own recording.
- Don't violate any ethical rules.
- Don't get emotional. Stay in control.
- Be confident and clear.
- Smile. Be Yourself.

Television or Skype Interview—What to Wear, Where to Look, and What to Say

If you are going to appear on television, you will want to learn a few tips. Things like what to wear and where to look when the camera is on may seem pretty basic but can make or break your appearance and impact. Dressing in professional business attire is usually recommended.

You want to be comfortable but make sure what you wear is conveying the image you want to project. Wear whatever you would wear in person to speak to an audience or for a professional interview. Follow whatever is the professional norm in your environment. Remember that it is usually better to be slightly overdressed than underdressed. It is a good idea to have a jacket lapel or shirt collar where a microphone can be attached. You can also consider bringing an additional jacket, suit, or dress in another color, just in case the one you are wearing does not work for some reason. Remember, your clothes and your appearance are your image and will make a statement.

Ask the reporters where you should look when you are talking and answering questions. They may want you to look directly at the camera or directly at them or at the audience if there is an audience present. Be comfortable and natural and know that your facial expressions will look best if you can just look directly into someone's eyes. If you must look into the camera lens, then imagine you are looking at a person. Relax and just answer the questions calmly, confidently, and as if you were talking to patients, medical students, or family members.

Clothes for On-Camera Appearance

- Professional business attire is usually best.
- Wear something that fits and is comfortable whether you stand or sit.
- Avoid wearing black or very dark clothing.
- Avoid wearing all white (a doctor's white coat is usually not good, but you can bring one as an option). White doesn't look good on camera.
- Avoid busy, loud prints or tiny prints or checkered clothing.
- Avoid large jewelry because it can cause noise.
- Have a suit, shirt, or dress lapel or collar to attach a microphone to.

- Do not wear hats or large earrings.
- Your hair should be clean and well-groomed.
- Wear dress shoes (assume your legs and feet will be seen).
- Blue suits with light shirts and tie look best on camera for men.
- Women can usually wear pastels or bright solid colors.
- Bring a backup suit or dress in case you need to change.

The reporter will tell you where to stand or sit and where to look. Make sure you are comfortable. Take a big deep breath. Smile if appropriate. You are the expert, and just imagine that you are speaking confidently and appropriately to a family member, friend, or a trusted colleague. If you are calm, then your face and your voice will be calm. Remember that you are the authority on the subject. Try to give brief answers and stick to the important points you wrote out before the interview. Answer the questions in a succinct and sincere manner. Think about how your voice, your words, and your body language are engaging the reporter. Be natural and conversational, and you will be informative.

Radio and Podcast Interviews

Radio interviews are similar to television interviews in that you will be speaking into a microphone and answering questions from a reporter. Sometimes you will be sitting across from the reporter, sometimes you may just listen to the reporter's voice through a phone line or ear piece. Or you may be sitting in a recording studio and will see the reporter through the glass in another studio. Of course, normally you will not be videotaped, but the more you can sit up and lean into the microphone and speak clearly and confidently, the better. Listen to the questions from the reporter and answer them. The more relaxed you are, the more relaxed your voice will be and the clearer your message will sound. You can imagine you are having a phone conversation. Make sure you are not wearing any jewelry or clothing that will make noise if you move your body in any way. Make sure you are comfortable, well-rested, and well-hydrated. Think of it as a conversation with your patients and the public. The information will usually be on a basic level. You might want to think about how clear and encouraging you are when you talk to a medical trainee or a patient while you are talking to the reporter. The reporter needs you to help the audience understand the information and can be thought of as the conduit for bringing your message to the public.

Press Conference—How to Handle Yourself

Most press conferences are convened by a hospital, university, or other institution because something has occurred that a lot of reporters want to know about. Instead of granting twenty separate interviews to twenty different reporters, a PR or communications person will usually convene a press conference at a specific time in a specific location. The topic can be good news, such as the opening of a new wing of the hospital or the successful outcome of a unique surgery. But it can also be bad news, such as an investigation into financial fraud, an alarming rate of hospital-acquired infections, or a large medical emergency in the community, such as a mass shooting, a fire, an earthquake, or an infectious disease outbreak.

If you are asked to be a speaker at a press conference, make sure to ask lots of questions of those organizing the press conference beforehand. Find out how many other speakers, if any, will be on the panel with you. Find out how many reporters will be there, what media organizations will be represented (e.g., television, newspaper) and what types of questions they might ask. Tell the organizers you want to walk through exactly how the press conference will run, including who will speak first and where the cameras and microphones will be located and how long it will last. Once the real press conference begins, always assume everything you say when you are in the room can be heard and is being recorded. Assume there are microphones and cameras and other recording devices on the entire time. Try to predict all of the questions the reporters may ask, positive and negative, on the topic. Write down your answers in two to three sentences with clear and simple statements. Prepare the most important points you want to make. Make sure you have accurate and up-to-date information and data. Find out how long you will have to speak. Ask if you will be making a "statement" first before taking questions. Ask if you can practice taking questions from your PR expert before the press conference begins. One way to learn about press conferences is by asking your PR person to allow you to attend one that you are not involved in; once there, you can just sit in the back row, watch, listen, and learn. Some institutions and communications training programs will run "mock press conferences" for their employees to learn, practice, and prepare before they are asked to appear and participate at a real press conference.

Writing Your Own Article

Have you always wanted to write a medical news or magazine article? Where do you start? How do you get it published? Just like when you submit an article to a medical journal, you need to be very familiar with the topics and style of articles that the particular newspaper or magazine publishes. You don't want to send a great news or opinion article you have written more suited for *The New Yorker Magazine* to *Reader's Digest,* or vice versa. You also don't want to pitch a story idea to your local newspaper if they just covered the issue recently and you have no new information to offer. If you want to publish in *The New York Times,* then you need to read *Science Times,* the health and science section, published every Tuesday. If you want to publish in your local newspaper or a national magazine, then look closely at the topics and the length of the articles. If your topic and your style of writing seems to fit there, then think about submitting your article. You can either "pitch a story idea" by writing a one paragraph synopsis or submit your entire article. Go to the website of any newspaper or magazine and look for the editor of that section's name and read the directions on how to submit your article. You can also consult Writers Market on how to get published.[6] This resource is published annually and updated with information from newspapers, magazines, and other venues for publication.

The most difficult step in writing a news story is finding a story idea. Many of my students and colleagues want to write articles and come to me discussing a myriad of people they would like to interview and issues that they would like to write about in their article, but when I ask them to tell me about their article in one sentence or to give me the title, they are dumbstruck. If you cannot describe your article in one sentence or articulate what the working title might be, then you may not have an idea for an article. A sentence describing your article is essentially your headline and should make your intended audience want to read the article. Sometimes you don't know what you want to write about because you haven't done enough research or reading or you haven't talked to enough people. Often journalists will set out to write one article but in going about researching the story through reading, data collection, and interviewing people, they find a better story to write than the initial one they were thinking about. When you have your idea for your article, remember that you still need to describe the story idea in one sentence.

Many physicians write their own articles because they want to tell the public what they find themselves saying daily to their patients, such as "make healthy lifestyle changes," "take your blood pressure medicine," or "follow these diabetes guidelines to help avoid complications." Some physician authors will act like reporters and interview many subjects (think Atul Gawande, author of "The Cost Conundrum: What a Texas Town Can Teach Us about Health Care" published in *The New Yorker Magazine*, June 1, 2009) that was read by many, including President Barack Obama. Other physicians will write articles based on their own expertise and not interview any other experts. You may be in either camp. You can always take a writing workshop or a journalism course to try to hone your skills.

You can also look at the myriad of resources about improving your writing from magazines and books to conferences and organizations. If you want to learn how to become a medical writer, you will likely need to learn and practice your skills before getting published. Many medical writers end up writing for biotechnology firms, pharmaceutical or medical device companies, or working in communications or advertising. Many physicians who want to write articles want to have their work published in the mainstream media. Here are some resources:

Resources for Writers

The Writer's Market: www.writersmarket.com
The Writer's Digest: http://www.writersdigest.com
American Medical Writers Association: https://
    www.amwa.org
National Association of Science Writers: https://
    www.nasw.org
Association of Health Care Journalists: https://
    healthjournalism.org
Nieman Reports (Nieman Foundation at Harvard University): https://niemanreports.org
Columbia Journalism Review (Columbia University School of Journalism): https://www.cjr.org

When you know the topic you want to write about, such as hypertension in the elderly, fear of vaccines, or the workings of your life as a clinical researcher, you next need to figure out who your audience is, outline the information and points you will express, and determine what type of article it will be (e.g., news, essay, opinion and perspective), what publication would be interested in the topic and your writing style, how long the article will be, and exactly how you will go about accomplishing your goal.

I often teach my medical students who want to be medical writers one important lesson: **the audience does not know as much as you do about your topic, nor do they care as much as you do. Your job is to teach them what you know and make them care about it.**

Tips for Writing Your Medical News Article Like a Journalist

1. Figure out what you want to write about. Find the topic that moves you, and you will move your audience.
2. Start thinking of as many questions as you can on your topic. In other words, figure out what you know and what you don't know—and most important, what you and your reader need to know.
3. Find the answers to your questions (as well as develop more questions) through interviews, reading, and data collection.
4. Be able to describe your article in one sentence.
5. Outline your article so that you know the structure and logical flow. How will the piece start and how will it end? What ground will you cover in the middle?
6. Teach your reader all that you know.
7. Tell your reader a story and make them care about the story as much as you do.

Writing an Op-Ed Article

Op-ed articles are opinion articles published on the editorial pages of newspapers. Newspapers publish op-ed articles written by members of the public because it not only broadens their editorial voice but also potentially increases the quality and quantity of the topics covered in their editorial section. People write op-eds generally because they have a strong opinion or interesting perspective on a topic of concern to the public. As a physician, you may want to write an op-ed article about a new research finding, a change in medicine guidelines, or an issue in healthcare delivery or reimbursement. You may want to recap new standards of care or send a message to your peers or to lawmakers. As a physician, you are in a unique position to write an editorial because of your perspective as well as your access to information, knowledge, and experience about important subjects that would be of interest to many. I have written several op-ed and other types of articles and perspectives on subjects ranging from food labels and end-of-life issues to bioterrorist threats and rising cholesterol levels in children. The following are some samples:

Smallpox Vaccination—A Call to Arms
by T. L. Schraeder and E. W. Campion
New England Journal of Medicine, January 30, 2003
The possibility of biologic warfare has entered the national psyche. Vaccination against smallpox has begun. For physicians and other healthcare professionals, the current call to arms means more than rolling up our sleeves for the prick of a bifurcated smallpox-vaccine needle. It means making sensitive decisions for ourselves and giving important education and advice to our patients. After all, we have faced fearful uncertainties before, and we do have wisdom from past experience.

Deteriorating Children's Health Isn't a Mystery
by Terry L. Schraeder
The Boston Globe, February 1, 2010
From anxiety and hormonal disorders to high blood pressure and type 2 diabetes, doctors are treating boys and girls for numerous medical conditions that were once uncommon or never seen in children—and many are preventable. Now we have one more to add to the list: high cholesterol. The Centers for Disease Control and Prevention recently released the following data for 1999–2006: one in five children aged 12–19 have high lipid levels (cholesterol or triglycerides) in their blood.

Weighing an Ounce of Healthcare Prevention
by Terry L. Schraeder
The Boston Globe, July 6, 2009
In all the ways the Obama administration and others are proposing to cut healthcare costs, including a single-payer option, limiting malpractice claims, and increased use and uniformity of electronic medical records, there is one that everyone—patients and doctors both—can utilize immediately: preventative health.

The medical system can no longer afford us the luxury of plopping down in front of our doctors and just saying "fix me."

Calorie Counts for Fast Foods
by Terry L. Schraeder
The Providence Journal, January 13, 2007
In December, New York City—known for its food as much as its fashion—passed two laws that attempt to make a difference in its residents' waistlines and mortality. The first passed by the City Health Department—and the most covered by the media—mandates that restaurants stop serving the partially hydrogenated oils that add shelf life to foods but remove life from us by clogging our arteries.

A Doctor's Take on Bioterrorism Fears: Don't Panic; Plan Ahead

by Terry L. Schraeder

The Boston Globe, October 2, 2001

A Boston-area doctor is confronted by a father with a sack of antibiotics. He wants to know if he has enough medication for his entire family in case of a bioterrorist attack. Neighbors and relatives call a critical-care doctor asking for medication in case anthrax is released. An infectious disease specialist reports the rapid unexplained death of a young woman to the Centers for Disease Control and Prevention—just to be sure he's not overlooking signs of bioterrorism. The fear of biological warfare is bordering on bio-hysteria.

Making Our Wishes Known

by Terry L. Schraeder

The Boston Globe, December 5, 2006

Many people in my generation are watching and worrying as our parents get further and further into their senior years. My own 75-year-old mother's health is slowly but certainly ebbing. Each week there seems to be a new health issue that needs attention: something on her body to be scoped, or biopsied, X-rayed, or MRI'd.

Doctors and Nurses Often Spread Flu, Rather than Stop It

by Terry L. Schraeder

The Boston Globe, October 5, 2004

What if a vaccine helped prevent hundreds of thousands of hospitalizations and 36,000 deaths in the United States each year? Certainly, all healthcare workers would roll up their sleeves to protect their patients and themselves, right? Wrong. According to the Centers for Disease Control and Prevention, only about one third of healthcare workers nationwide receive a flu vaccination each year.

First, and most important, you will want to figure out the reason you are writing the op-ed or other type of news article. Are you trying to inform the public on an important medical topic such as a rise in infectious diseases or suicide rates? Are you trying to share your perspective on a provocative topic in the news such as lethal injections or abortion? Are you trying to highlight your unique voice on a subject such as the death of the solo practice or rise in physician burnout?

You will also want to figure out who your audience is. Who do you want to read your article: your peers, your patients, or the public? Why would they be interested in your article? Are you trying to send a message to healthcare executives, insurance agencies, or government officials? After you figure out who you are writing the article to, you can tailor the message and the information for them. But you must remember that you will also need to convince an editor to publish your op-ed. An editor will determine if the topic and the message are of interest and relevant to their readership and if your writing is clear and informative. Pat Skerrett, Editor of *First Opinion*, manages the op-ed section for the online media organization, STAT. He believes the op-ed must past the "Wow!" factor or the "Hmm" test to get past the editor. He also believes that your article needs to contain not just your opinion but "rock solid facts" to educate the reader. He believes in the 80-20 rule: you need 80% new information and 20% opinion in your op-ed article, particularly if you have no particular expertise or name recognition.

The best way to figure out how to write an op-ed article is to read as many editorials and op-ed articles in your newspaper as you can. See how the writers grab the reader with a strong opening sentence or paragraph and then use interesting and accurate information to support their arguments and main points. Learn how they incorporate a "call to action" and leave the readers with a concluding "take-away" message. Try to emulate these published editorials in your own conversational voice. Use your authority and knowledge but also be willing to share your personal story and message.

Remember to review the guidelines of submitting such an opinion article on the newspaper's website. Op-ed articles are usually less than 800 words and some less than 500 words. Try to write in an active voice and avoid the passive voice. In an active voice, the subject performs the action. In a passive voice, the subject receives the action.

> **Passive:** Diabetes complications are related to a poor diet and poor management of blood sugar.
>
> **Active:** A poor diet and poor management of blood sugar can lead to complications for diabetics.
>
> **Passive:** Opioid addiction is related to the misuse of legally prescribed narcotics.
>
> **Active:** The misuse of prescription narcotics can lead to opioid addiction.
>
> **Passive:** Obesity is influenced by long hours of computer screen time and intake of high-calorie foods.
>
> **Active:** Long hours of computer screen time and intake of high-calorie foods promote obesity.

Becoming a "Source"

Another way to engage with the press is to become a source. If your expertise is in cardiology or orthopedics, you can always introduce yourself and send your contact information and credentials to a journalist and offer to be a source when your expertise is needed. If you see a story in the newspaper regarding an area you know about, send an email or note to the reporter saying you would be available if the reporter ever writes about this subject again. The best way to start a relationship with a journalist is to contact the writer with a new story idea, such as the rise in the rate of hip replacements in middle-aged patients or another topic that has not been publicized or explained in the lay press.

You can also offer them new sources including names of experts in the field, journals, organizations and medical conferences regarding a medical news story they are interested in. Reporters and editors need new story ideas and new sources. They don't necessarily need more physicians who think they're writers. If you do have a new story idea, then by all means contact a reporter or write the article yourself. If you learn about an interesting new finding or witness a trend in medicine you think would be of interest to the public, or want to share your own published research (and you can make it understandable and relevant to the public), then a journalist would love to hear from you.

Conversely, if you do read an article in your local newspaper that you think was incomplete or inaccurate, you can always contact the reporter or the editor and offer to provide your insight and expertise on what the article was missing. If you do this in a polite and informative manner, usually the journalist will want to hear more from you. Or you can write a letter to the editor, which if accepted will put your name and message into the pages of the newspaper on the subject. Of course, most papers now allow for online comments on their websites or through their social media websites as well—this is another way to get your name, expertise, and opinion noticed and acknowledged.

Journalists and editors need story ideas and new information. They also need people who can translate complex topics and engage the public. If you can do this, they will be interested in knowing you and hiring you (or at least publishing your article).

Chasm of Distrust in Medical Journalism

Whatever your feelings are about the press in general and whether you decide to interact with the media or not, there are a few important points to remember. Several years ago, I was struck by the chasm of distrust that had developed between physicians and journalists, so I wrote the following article for the *Nieman Reports* at the Nieman Foundation at Harvard University:

A Chasm of Distrust in Medical Reporting

by Terry L. Schraeder, MD (*Nieman Reports;* Nieman Foundation at Harvard; June 15, 2003; https://niemanreports.org/articles/a-chasm-of-distrust-in-medical-reporting/)

After working as a medical journalist for 10 years, I entered medical school and then a residency in internal medicine. To my surprise, I emerged to find a new world of medical journalism. I am encouraged by some aspects of this world but disillusioned by others. It is true that medical journalism, more than ever before, has become an important source of public health education and information. But it is also true that there are problems in the relationship between medical journalists and physicians, including their understanding of each other's professions.

The chasm between medical journalists and physicians appears mostly to be one of ignorance rather than conflicting interests or malice. But across this divide exist miscommunication, misunderstanding and the potential for misguided messages to the public. Rose-colored glasses may have altered my memory, but I do not recall the caustic attitudes of journalists toward doctors or the skeptical tenor of doctors toward journalists when I was a full-time journalist a decade ago. I remember more professional respect, objective analysis, and collaboration. Perhaps, during the embryonic years of mainstream medical journalism, the parties were more polite, if not forgiving and patient of each other.

The worsening rift first struck me after I finished my medical internship. Working as a freelance journalist, I thought I would be welcomed back into the fold of the fourth estate. Instead, I felt like an outsider. Negative comments about the medical profession seemed commonplace. Likewise, I heard physicians speak of members of the press as if they were not to be trusted.

I listened to routine condemnation of medicine and journalism often framed with incomplete or inaccurate data. Instead of talking about story ideas and interesting science and medicine, journalists railed and postured as if they were protecting the public from a menace. It was as if in covering medicine, they were covering the enemy. Physicians dismissed medical journalists as being too uneducated to understand medicine or too busy to report on it accurately. They worried about the limitations of journalists and the motives of their editors while pointing to manipulation by outside interests. News reports were considered "abbreviated" at best and "sensational" at worst. Doctors accused the media of confusing their patients.

For me, the dispute came into focus at the Mayo Clinic's Medicine and Media Conference in 2002. One reporter charged that if journalists had not reported on the limitations of arthroscopic surgery that doctors would not have changed their practice of performing arthroscopy for osteoarthritis of the knee.

The journalist in me wanted to say, "Yes, mainstream medical journalists covered that research and informed the public." But the doctor in me wanted to say, "Doctors designed and conducted that research and a medical journal (*The New England Journal of Medicine,* July 11, 2002) published the study showing that arthroscopic surgery has no benefit over placebo for the treatment of certain types of osteoarthritis of the knee." A change in practice came about because of a collaborative effort instituted by doctors and conveyed to the lay public by journalists.

I began to wonder whether journalists and doctors are oblivious to the importance of their collaboration. And I worried that the negative attitudes they had about one another could threaten similar effective working relationships of the future. Had medicine become the enemy, as some medical journalists thought? Are most medical journalists unable to inform and educate the public accurately on important health matters, as some physicians believed?

In trying to answer these questions, I thought of numerous examples of outstanding work from both fields. In my journey of medical reporting and medical training, I've witnessed countless instances of commitment, intelligence, and courage from physicians and medical journalists, all working under profound professional stresses. So why the cynical attitudes toward one another?

What to Do about Distrust

No one will dispute the fact that the problems in medicine are vast, from the economic implosion affecting the ability of the profession to fulfill its mission to the limitations of the system to handle all aspects of medical care. Few disagree about the crisis of medical errors or the critical need to improve medical training and health care delivery especially for our aging and poor populations. But journalists and physicians working independently or as adversaries will not solve these problems.

Similarly, most would recognize that medical journalists are under enormous constraints of time, space and background knowledge. Many must cover an unimaginable range of complex medical topics on a day-to-day basis. Journalists must place an inordinate trust in their sources and constantly worry about both missing some aspect of the story and the health implications of informing the public about medicine. Their beat is a moving target, where scientific interpretations and health recommendations change often.

Do doctors and journalists have a responsibility to work together? Can and should they develop a cohesive system to educate and inform the public as well as keep an eye on each other? Shouldn't they recognize that they share many of the same frustrations and restrictions, as well as ideals and goals? These issues—and others—must be articulated in an intelligent and constructive debate among individuals who have not lost respect for either profession. We must hear from those who will propose and implement effective solutions.

One example of a medical situation that would greatly benefit from collaborative trust and better communication is the diversion of ambulances from hospitals because of overcrowded emergency rooms. This is an important story, but most of the coverage of this issue has not included those inside medicine or public health who could help uncover and explain why the problem exists. Both the complexity and the magnitude of the story were missed. Furthermore, the reactionary "solutions" made by some hospitals in response to newspaper headlines were worse than the original problem. Overwhelmed and understaffed emergency rooms are not better for patients than hospital diversions.

At times, the relationship between doctors and journalists resembles a bad marriage, with equal parts dependence and disdain. Neither group seems to understand nor acknowledge the other's roles and responsibilities. Ultimately, the public and patients suffer. Perhaps those in medicine who criticize journalists for misleading the public might move away from providing only criticism and begin to find more effective means of improving communication or providing technical assistance to journalists. Whether it is books on epidemiology, symposia on infectious diseases, or other professional development workshops, journalists would welcome the information. Furthermore, for doctors to relinquish the job of public health education and place it solely in the hands of the mainstream press is neither fair nor prudent.

Also, during the Mayo Clinic meeting, one speaker implied that if the press had not covered the hormone replacement study last summer, many gynecologists would not have called their patients or changed their prescribing practices. The hormone replacement study was released in a major medical journal (*The Journal of the American Medical Association*, July 2002) that is read by physicians and journalists. Such peer-reviewed journals help to set policy and practice standards. Whether the mass media covered the hormone story or not, most agree that medical practice would have changed and patients would have been notified.

Although many important stories are covered in the mainstream press, medicine is not taught in a 30-second sound bite, nor does it generally change on the basis of a newspaper headline. With the hormone replacement study, the media helped get the word to patients but, unfortunately, the complex conclusions of the message and the way it was released might have caused more confusion. If physicians and members of the media had collaborated on how best to get this message to patients and physicians—as suggested in an article, "Menopausal Hormone Therapy: Summary of a Scientific Workshop," published in the *Annals of Internal Medicine* (February 18, 2003), everyone might have readily benefited.

Bridging the Chasm

Doctors and medical journalists both define themselves as public servants. They come together at a crossroads of public health. If they are to be patient advocates, they cannot be arch antagonists. They must fulfill their responsibilities to the public through professional cooperation and mutual understanding.

I am not suggesting that they be "yes men" or that they not expose one another's fallibilities and mistakes. But I do think it best if each becomes knowledgeable about the other's profession, whether guarding against medical errors in the hospital or in the headlines. This won't happen if each does not understand the other's professional training, education, deadlines, responsibilities, codes of ethics, and internal stresses.

Several years ago, I was speaking at a national health journalism conference when a journalist in the audience suggested how counterintuitive it was that a researcher would write a hypothesis before conducting a study and interpreting data. I knew that to do otherwise would be anathema to reputable research. Conversely, to explain to a doctor or clinical scientist why a journalist would never write a headline before they wrote their story might seem odd. Furthermore, to try to explain how a journalist could set out to write one story but then return to their editor with another would be difficult. It might appear even suspect.

Given today's realities of covering medical news, an important genetic discovery of a lethal disease often needs to be communicated in one-and-a-half minutes or 500 words. There is much at stake in journalists being sure this difficult job is done well since both patients and practitioners have come to rely upon medical journalism to help stay informed.

I must admit that I have heard more criticism from journalists of doctors than doctors of journalists. Of course, this might be related to the nature of a journalist's work; after all, medical journalists encounter doctors and cover the medical profession nearly every day. Most doctors come into contact with journalists on an irregular basis, if at all.

How are physicians affected by medical journalism? I am completing a research project that assesses physicians' attitudes about the news media and how medical information in the popular press affects them, their patients, and their practices. I also hope to help these two professions better understand each other. Perhaps my study will facilitate an intelligent and productive discourse between doctors and journalists.

I know firsthand of the promises of both professions. I do not want the current adversarial abyss that lies between them to threaten their potential or harm their work. While keeping our roles and responsibilities distinct and clear, we must begin to build a bridge over the chasm. Only then, will we as doctors and medical journalists truly serve the public and our professions.

I still feel the same way I did when I first wrote this article. Today, more than ever before, I believe our patients, the public, and the profession of medicine all benefit when we improve our communications skills as physicians and consider engaging with the press and the public at large.

Further Reading

American Medical Association, Press Release, "AMA Adopts Guidance for Ethical Physician Conduct in the Media," November 14, 2017.

American Medical Association, Ethical Physician Conduct in the Media, Code of Medical Ethics Opinion 8.2. Retrieved from: https://www.ama-assn.org/delivering-care/ethics/ethical-physician-conduct-media.

Susan Dentzer, "Communicating Medical News—Pitfalls of Health Care Journalism," *New England Journal of Medicine*, 2009; 360:1–3, doi: 10.1056/NEJMp0805753EJM.

Heidi Moawad, "How Doctors Can Communicate with the Media," *MD Magazine*, August 15, 2018. Retrieved from: https://www.mdmag.com/physicians-money-digest/practice-management/how-doctors-can-connect-with-the-media.

References

1. American Medical Association: Ethical Physician Conduct in the Media, Code of Medical Ethics Opinion 8.2. Retrieved from: https://www.ama-assn.org/delivering-care/ethics/ethical-physician-conduct-media.

2. Institutes of Medicine, Committee on Assuring the Health of the Public in the 21st Century, *The Future of the Public's Health in the 21st Century* (Washington, DC: National Academies Press, 2002).

3. J. Laugesen, K. Hassanein, and Y. Yuan, "The Impact of Internet Health Information on Patient Compliance: A Research Model and an Empirical Study," *Journal of Medical Internet Research*, 2015;17(6):e143, doi: 10.2196/jmir.4333.

4. X. Liang, L. Y.-F. Su, S. K. Yeo et al., "Building Buzz: (Scientists) Communicating Science in New Media Environments," *Journalism and Mass Communication Quarterly*, 2014;91(4):772–791, doi: 10.1177/1077699014550092.

5. J. B. Nie, A. Gilbertson, M. de Roubaix et al., "Healing without Waging War: Beyond Military Metaphors in Medicine and HIV Cure Research," *American Journal of Bioethics*, 2016;16(10):3–11. Retrieved from: https://www.ncbi.nlm.nih.gov/pmc/articles/PMC5064845/.

6. *Writer's Market 2019: The Most Trusted Guide to Getting Published*, 98th edition (Cincinnati, OH: Writer's Digest Books, 2018). Retrieved from: http://www.writersmarket.com.

Index

preparation for talking to, 176–77, 179, 184–86, 189–90
reasons for talking to, 174–78
reasons to engage with the media as a physician, 168
using caution when talking to, 184–86
medical information, 109
in popular media, 172–73
privacy of personal (*see* privacy; protected health information)
in social media, 61–62, 64, 71–75, 80–82
medical news. *See* news
medical students/medical trainees, teaching communication skills to, 45–47
advice for, 50–51
questions to ask yourself while students and resident follow you, 48–50
medicine, five pillars for the practice of, 2–3
metaphors
defined, 177
military, 38–39, 177
use of, 176–78
microphone, 128, 162, 164, 188–90
military metaphors, 38–39, 177
"ministry of presence," 35, 84
mission, xix–xx. *See also* MACY
knowing your, xix–xx, 147
mistakes, fear of making, 140
monotone voice, fear of speaking in, 141
Mukherjee, Siddhartha, 70
mumbling, 125. *See also* articulation

Nerurkar, Aditi, 72
nervous energy, channeling, 138
nervousness when speaking, 121, 122, 124, 127
emergency toolbox for, 140–42
letting your nerves get the best of you, 137–43

realizing when it is normal to be nervous, 137–38
Neuendorf, Katie, 12
New England Journal of Medicine (NEJM), 173
social media and, 66–69, 67f, 80
Terry Schraeder and, xviii, 167, 171, 172
news, medical. *See also under* writing
survey of physicians on the impact of, 172–74
news media. *See* media
nonverbal communication, 41–42
Noonan, Peggy, 156

Obamacare (Affordable Care Act), xvii, 9
observational learning, 45–46
observing natural communicators, 149–50
"off the record," 182, 185, 186
on-camera appearance. *See also* television interviews
clothes for, 161–62
on-camera presentations. *See also* video presentations
delivery, 160
video skills, 158–61
"on the record," 182, 185
op-ed articles, 194, 197–98
sample articles, 194–96
Osler, William, 23b

passive vs. active voice, 197–98
pathos. *See* rhetorical triangle
patience, 30–31
patient portals, 106–8
patient portal visits, 107–8
Patient Protection and Affordable Care Act, xvii, 9
patients. *See also specific topics*
letting them tell their story, 20–23b
need to regain their agency, 7
what they want, 18–19
patient satisfaction, 13, 19, 50
patient satisfaction surveys, 9–10

214   INDEX